Evaluating HIV
Prevention Interventions

AIDS Prevention and Mental Health

Series Editors:

David G. Ostrow, M.D., Ph.D.
Howard Brown Health Center and Illinois Masonic Medical Center, Chicago, Illinois

Jeffrey A. Kelly, Ph.D.
Medical College of Wisconsin, Milwaukee, Wisconsin

A Continuation Order Plan is available for this series. A continuation order will bring delivery of each new volume immediately upon publication. Volumes are billed only upon actual shipment. For further information please contact the publisher.

Foreword

In 1985 Gay Men's Health Crisis (GMHC) of New York City, was awarded one of the very earliest federally sponsored HIV prevention programs. Evaluation was central to the GMHC effort—essentially because the entire nation knew next to nothing about what would work for HIV prevention. The Centers for Disease Control (CDC) faced major political barriers in funding the GMHC project along with a very small number of other HIV prevention projects. GMHC, along with those other projects, fought substantial delays, opposition from the radical right, and the threat of defunding from the Reagan White House. Only a handful of prevention researchers were interested in HIV at the time—perhaps it bore a stigma.

Yet those first demonstration studies were invaluable to the nation as it began to understand how to stop the spread of the epidemic. Equally impressive, the evaluation of the GMHC project was informative and useful for the organization itself, enabling it to finetune its prevention efforts.

Three lessons are driven home by GMHC's experience with this early evaluation. The lessons need to be taken to heart by AIDS services organizations, health departments, and other prevention agencies everywhere. The first lesson is: you can do useful evaluation. The authors of this book faced many prevention and evaluation challenges both before and after this episode, with and without government funding, and with and without a variety of other constraints. They moved on to other positions in government and the private sector, but always with a focus on AIDS prevention and treatment. This book demystifies evaluation for the practitioner. Without departing from best practice in evaluation, it gives practitioners and researchers the specific tools that have proven useful in HIV prevention.

The second lesson is: evaluation can improve practice. This book provides abundant examples that are directly applicable even to the most modest prevention effort. Particularly helpful is the focus on understanding the logic of program delivery, since the unique considerations for HIV prevention programs (such as outreach to populations that are not commonly seen in medical care settings) carry over into important considerations for evaluation. Also helpful are comments on applying behavioral theories to HIV prevention. Theory behind the programs has become recognized as central to guiding evaluation methods (Chen, 1990; Lipsey, 1993). Not enough good examples of specific prevention application are available (Leviton, 1989; 1996). Application is not simple or straightforward; if it were, many more good models of HIV prevention would be available than we have at present (Leviton & O'Reilly, 1996). Guidance on program development can be informed by evaluation, and this book illustrates the process very well.

The book contains a variety of examples on an international scale. The authors have gone beyond the published literature from the epicenter's study of the usual suspects. Prevention interventions from around the globe are included. In addition to a summary of the program content, evaluation approaches are outlined. There is something for every program developer and evaluator in many areas of HIV prevention in a variety of geographic locales. Further, this volume reports on the activities of projects that have multiple funding sources.

The need for good models is every bit as pressing as it was when the original prevention projects were conducted. Only good evaluation can help us to improve these models. Kelly, Murphy, Sikkema, and Kalichman said it succinctly, "After more than 12 years of the HIV epidemic—an epidemic that can only be controlled by interventions to promote risk behavior change—the lack of research evaluating outcomes of interventions to prevent HIV infection is very troubling" (1993, p. 1025). Prevention at its best has still only chipped away at the margins of an overwhelming epidemic. Unlike other volumes, this book focuses on the merging of theory and practice as a means to fully evaluate an intervention. This merger puts the theoretical into the hands of the frontline user.

This brings me to the third lesson from the authors' experience: no excuses—we need evaluations of your programs. The field of HIV prevention still needs to know what works, and needs to study it scientifically. Evaluations do not have to involve highly expensive research methods or the most rigorous scientific designs to be informative. We should strive for rigor to get the best answers—rigor is not necessarily expensive. But evaluations can be useful even when they are not perfect. For many aspects of program design, it will be more important to share imperfect knowledge than to wait for some vague future in which all is revealed about how to prevent HIV. Vulnerable populations cannot wait for that future.

We still need improvements in HIV prevention program evaluation; and we need them from practitioners as well as behavioral scientists. Practitioners will have adapted good ideas to a variety of settings, many populations, and organizations constrained both by expertise and finances. They will often be more concerned with what is practical and cost-effective. The researchers have not cornered the market on good ideas. Far from it. Nor should they corner the market on evaluation.

Practitioners sometimes hesitate to conduct evaluation because they are so busy doing—they may not feel there is time or priority for reflecting on how they are doing. The authors of this book will, I believe, persuade HIV prevention programs that there are real advantages to the process of pausing to reflect.

Laura C. Leviton, Ph.D.
Professor, University of Alabama at Birmingham,
School of Public Health

Preface

In designing, implementing, and evaluating HIV risk-reduction interventions in 1986, we were frequently called on to assist others in developing evaluation methodologies for their programs. We quickly realized that few community-based organizations or governmental agencies were conducting evaluations; there were limited models reported in the literature; there was a lot to learn about this type of evaluation; and we did not have all the answers. The seed for this volume was planted in late 1988 as we began to search for a way to share our experiences in developing and evaluating innovative HIV prevention programs. The need to make these successes and failures known to other community-based organizations was recognized by Dr. Charles E. McKinney, then Gay Men's Health Crisis (GMHC) director of education, whose foresight, support, and encouragement were catalysts to the "birth" of this volume.

The HIV epidemic presents a number of ethical dilemmas for researchers conducting behavioral interventions and evaluations, epidemiological, psychosocial, clinical, and basic research studies. Of major debate is how to conduct research in which the quality and integrity of the research are preserved without compromising the confidentiality of the participants. Results of behavioral research studies may have far-reaching effects, especially when used as a basis to formulate and shape public policy (Grodin, Kaminow & Sassower, 1986). Therefore, evaluation needs to be valid and reliable, built on the expertise of social scientists and public health specialists, as well as on the theories that they have developed and tested.

The issues raised in this volume are relevant to the evaluation of public health prevention programs in general. There is no evaluation methodology specific to AIDS, per se. This book integrates evaluation within the context of HIV preventive interventions; it translates evaluation and methodological jargon to program staff in community-based and nongovernmental organizations and professionals-in-training who may have had little or no formal preparation for program evaluation. It is also intended to help program administrators improve their programs and researchers enhance the quality of the evaluation data. Consequently, many examples are provided to illustrate points about methods and measurement. Developed to demonstrate the need for program evaluation, this volume incorporates the academic tenets of evaluation with their practical applications based on worldwide experiences. The text is liberally illustrated using tables, figures, examples, and case studies.

Overall, the evaluator may be involved in program planning as well as evaluation. He or she works with the sponsoring organization and community from the beginning of the program development. So, for each goal and objective, there is a simultaneous description of the evaluation questions and mechanisms (e.g., questionnaires, focus groups), as well as the personnel, equipment, and money necessary to evaluate the program successfully.

An early version of this publication was sent to an outside panel of experts noted in the Acknowledgments; their comments have been incorporated into this version of the volume. Since its initial review in 1989, the volume's scope broadened, its length more than tripled, and its target audience expanded. Its contents go beyond our experiences at GMHC. It includes our behavioral research and intervention experiences derived from the federally funded GMHC behavioral research program as well as those of many colleagues. Experience with varied target populations, prevention initiatives, and program evaluation techniques has sharpened our perspective of the problems faced by evaluators of HIV preventive interventions for community-based organizations, health departments, and other agencies.

This volume can be used as a springboard for new programming ideas as well as a reference to other sources in the published and unpublished literature. Its unique aspects, which add to its strength and usefulness, are an emphasis on the role of the community in the development, implementation, and evaluation of HIV/AIDS preventive interventions; recognition of the importance of quantitative and qualitative evaluation; application of 12 major public health theories/models; and descriptions of programs and evaluation results.

We believe this volume will help a wide range of readers appreciate the need for evaluating their HIV preventive interventions. The volume provides a concrete grounding in procedures, documentation and measurement, analysis, reporting, publishing, and dissemination of results. For the experienced researcher, it will assist in the development and evaluation of an intervention. For the less experienced, it sensitizes program staff to the need for evaluation and provides a useful reference tool.

Joanne E. Mantell
Anthony T. DiVittis
Marilyn I. Auerbach

Acknowledgments

Suggestions from numerous reviewers have been incorporated into this book. Any lack or faults are those of the authors, however. Reviewers who generously gave of their time to provide comments on this book were: Mitchell Cohen, PhD, Independent Consultant, New York, NY; Laura Leviton, PhD, Professor, University of Alabama, School of Public Health, Birmingham, AL; Michael Helquist, formerly Programme Officer, AIDSCOM Project, Academy for Educational Development, Washington, DC; Dorothy J. Jessop, PhD, Director of Research and Evaluation, Medical and Health Research Association of New York City, Inc.; Catherine Nelson, PhD, Deputy Director of Research and Evaluation, Medical and Health Research Association of New York City, Inc.; Annette Ramirez de Arellano, DrPH, Executive Director, Hispanic AIDS Forum, New York, NY; Lee Sechrest, PhD, Professor of Psychology, University of Arizona, Department of Psychology, Tucson, AZ; Patricia Webb, MA, Former Executive Director, Health Services Improvement Fund, New York, NY; and Karen Wyche, PhD, Associate Professor, School of Social Work, New York University, New York, NY.

Other colleagues reviewed specific chapters. Our thanks to Karen Denard Goldman, MPH, PhD, Assistant Professor, Department of Urban Studies and Community Health, Rutgers University, New Brunswick, NJ; Claire Jagemann, MPH, Director of Support Services for HIV Counseling and Testing, New York City Department of Health; and James M. Holmes, MPH, Instructor, Community Health Education Program, Hunter College School of Health Sciences, City University of New York, New York, NY.

Special thanks are also due to Robert F. Boruch, PhD, Department of Sociology, University of Pennsylvania, for directing us to key literature resources. Marie Tomlinson, MLS, a librarian at the Hunter College Health Professions Library, greatly assisted us in finding pertinent journals and books. Original artwork was generously contributed by Barbara Boer Rowes.

We would also like to acknowledge the late Charles E. McKinney, EdD, former Director of the Education Department at GMHC, for his support of the research programs and foresight in recognizing the need to disseminate information about GMHC's and other agencies' HIV preventive interventions and how to evaluate them. Funds for the development of the earlier version of this volume were provided by the Department of Education, GMHC.

Many of the ideas in this volume represent the collective work of other members of the GMHC Education and Research and Evaluation staff who generously committed their time beyond the expected call of duty to support our efforts to complete this volume. In particular, we acknowledge the efforts of Robin Lin Miller, PhD, formerly Director of Evaluation Research; Steven Humes, MPH, formerly Director of Prevention and Training; the late David Austin, formerly Assistant Director of Education; Andy Grogan, formerly Administrative Assistant; and Ann Podolske, Research Assistant.

Special thanks are also due to Anke A. Ehrhardt, PhD, Director, and Zena Stein, MB, BCh, Co-Director, HIV Center for Clinical and Behavioral Studies at the New York State Psychiatric Institute, and to members of the Center's Psychosocial/Qualitative Assessment Core: Susan E. Tross, PhD, Bruce D. Rapkin, PhD, Blanca Ortíz-Torres, JD, Lucile Newman, PhD, Karen Wyche, PhD, Sutherland Miller, PhD, and Robert Klitzman, MD.

Finally, we would like to thank our family and friends for their support and endurance. Special thanks to Lester J. Mantell, Pearl Benoliel, Phyliss Mantell, John Anspach, Dr. Arthur and Mrs. Loaettis DiVittis, Dr. Ann Brandwein, the Napolitano family, Evelyn and Rubin Auerbach, and the Chilibean family.

Contents

THE SOCIAL AND POLITICAL CONTEXTS OF EVALUATION

The feasibility and cost of an evaluation strategy and ability to answer questions about an intervention in a timely fashion need to be considered. For example, evaluations that involve longitudinal assessment of program impact, such as participants' maintenance of HIV-related risk-reduction behaviors or longer-term emotional responses to HIV testing, present a unique set of issues. Researchers need to assess whether changes in outcomes are due specifically to the intervention or to extraneous factors, such as increased media exposure about condoms or a celebrity figure's public announcement of his or her HIV infection. In addition, evaluators must deal with problems of subject attrition over time. While prolonged measurement enhances utility of the data gathered, it is costly and requires that agencies dedicate intensive resources to this endeavor. Before conducting costly large-scale studies, researchers should consider developing and evaluating a demonstration project in which the feasibility of a program is tested out on a small group from the target population, and, if proven effective, later replicated with a larger group of individuals.

More recently, there have been calls to include a cost analysis in the evaluation of HIV prevention programs (Choi & Coates, 1994; Holtgrave, 1994). Policymakers want to know whether program benefits outweigh program costs. This is especially important to CBOs in determining which programs on a cost and benefit basis are worthy of replicating (Holtgrave, 1994). Concern about the proper balance of monies expended for AIDS compared to other diseases has been a recurring issue (Pear, 1992) and is reflected in Senator Jesse Helms' call for a reduction in the amount of federal spending on AIDS (Dunlap, 1995).

These questions are obviously political. The best answer to critics of these programs is to prove their cost-effectiveness through program evaluation. Without this, accountability to funders and program participants cannot be accomplished, the ability to identify successful strategies and programs for behavioral change will be impeded, and limited resources will be wasted on untested interventions. Consequently, federal, state, and local government funders have increasingly recognized the need for evaluation (US General Accounting Office, 1988; New York State Department of Health AIDS Institute, 1994). Components of an intervention can be analyzed by actual use of material resources (e.g., condoms, brochures, diaries), participant incentives, staff and volunteer labor (in hours), and indirect costs (Holtgrave, 1994).

The stigmatization of and discrimination toward people with HIV infection have elevated levels of anxiety about the consequences of potential violations of confidentiality and have affected the conduct of HIV/AIDS research, including program evaluation (Melton & Gray, 1988; Walkey, Taylor, & Green, 1990). Safeguards to protect research participants' confidentiality and/or anonymity have resulted in the design of elaborate coding systems that conceal personal identifiers for data linkage (Bharucha-Reid, Schork, & Schwartz, 1990). Sometimes, the desire for anonymity has driven study design selection, e.g., the use of a cross-sectional (a study in which data are gathered at one point in time only) rather than a panel design (a study in which data are collected from the same persons over multiple time points). Because participants are not followed over time, their participation can be anonymous.

Due to historical medical exploitation, such as the Tuskegee syphilis experiments, in which poor black men infected with syphilis were denied diagnosis and standard treatment, ethnic minority groups may think twice before consenting to participate in research programs (Wilkerson, 1991; Thomas & Quinn, 1991; Jones, 1993). This distrust is further fueled by perceptions of a conspiracy theory—that HIV was unleashed by whites for the purpose of genocide of people of color.

THE NEED FOR CULTURAL SENSITIVITY

All evaluations should be undertaken with sensitivity to the subject matter and target population. However, when the focus is AIDS, awareness of the potential for stigma due to racism, gender, drug use, and sexual orientation is critical. Developers of HIV prevention programs attempt to deliver culturally sensitive, language-appropriate curriculum by credible sources. Programs must be acceptable and not perceived to be offensive by those groups for which they have been designed. Programs not tailored to a target group could well have little or no effect. Such failures occur because a program is thought to be irrelevant or inappropriate to the individual or community. It is unrealistic to assume that a generic prevention program will have a beneficial impact on diverse at-risk populations (Freudenberg, 1990). Just as we have learned that preventive health behaviors are not unidimensional, we have accepted that "one size fits all" interventions are unreasonable. Instead, selected content, activities, and teaching methods must be adapted to be population-specific.

ASSESSING ORGANIZATIONAL COMMITMENT

While there may be a need for evaluation, a first step is to determine whether an agency is committed to evaluating its HIV prevention program. Does management really want to know whether their safer sex workshop, HIV risk-reduction counseling, or outreach worker team efforts are effective prevention strategies? Prior to developing an evaluation strategy, there must be a clear understanding of how and by whom information derived from the evaluation will be used. Will the agency seek to constrain negative information about the program? Agency support and sanction of the program evaluation are essential, regardless of whether the evaluation is conducted by in-house staff or contracted outside. Of equal importance are an agency's trust and confidence in the evaluator, especially his or her ability to protect the privacy and confidentiality of information disclosed by program participants (Boruch, 1988b). This is also important from a participant's perspective, whether HIV-infected or not; assurance of safety from public disclosure, discrimination, and other possible reprisals can serve to increase program enrollment and retention rates. Institutional review boards (IRBs), long mandated by the federal government's Office of Protection of Research Risks in universities, hospitals, and other health agencies conducting research, are increasingly being set up by CBOs. The IRB is designed to safeguard the rights of research participants.

CBOs may be concerned that a formal program evaluation might reveal that their

AIDS preventive intervention had limited or no effect on changing participants' HIV-related knowledge, attitudes, and behaviors. This may occur even when an evaluation plan is carefully designed. Such findings might lead an administrator to conclude that program support should be withdrawn. Such "no difference" research, however, may provide useful lessons in how to improve research techniques and strengthen the design of evaluation strategies (Yeaton & Sechrest, 1987).

A CBO's reticence to be involved in evaluation research is often connected to a belief that it is costly and complicated. Before any organization engages in highly technical research designs, quasi-experimentation, and costly statistical analysis, it is important that the organization commits to formative evaluation strategies, such as implementation evaluation. The need to understand how a program was developed, how it meets the needs of its constituency, and the replicability of its design are essential features of program evaluation that can be implemented at low cost by the CBO (Miller & Cassel, in press).

DISSEMINATION OF EVALUATION RESULTS

The development, implementation, and evaluation of HIV preventive interventions are the three components most discussed in HIV/AIDS prevention. This volume also focuses on a fourth component: dissemination of research findings. By sharing information with the immediate circle involved in the intervention (e.g., the community, funders, and sponsoring organization), the bond between research and intervention is strengthened. But this is only one phase of dissemination. There is an unmet need to publish evaluation results for the caregiving communities.

Publication has many venues. Aside from articles in refereed journals and participation in professional conferences, other effective means of dissemination exist. Developing networks of health care professionals, mailing a quarterly newsletter (Martin, 1985), using computer bulletin boards, and convening organization-sponsored conferences all can be used to share information about the efficacy of intervention strategies.

Through the sharing of results, new intervention strategies can be developed at lower costs and program developers can be spared implementing ineffective evaluation strategies. The dissemination of evaluation results is even being included as a contract deliverable by funders in some awards (R. Duffy, 1995, personal communication).

The authors view dissemination of evaluation results as an obligation on the part of program designers and evaluators. Publication, in any form, completes the circle of the evaluation process.

SCOPE AND BLUEPRINT OF THIS VOLUME

This volume examines the evaluation of HIV preventive interventions designed to reduce HIV risks and therefore focuses on knowledge, attitude, and behavioral change. Therefore, evaluation of preventive interventions directed at clinical prophylaxis, including the safety of the nation's blood supply through donor testing, antiviral treatment, combination therapies such as protease inhibitors, and treatment for addiction and sexually transmitted diseases, and psychosocial interventions (e.g., anticipatory grief and bereavement, coping strategies with the disease), is outside the scope of this volume.

Evaluation methods cannot be discussed without addressing program development and implementation and how evaluation informs and strengthens all aspects of interventions. For HIV behavioral intervention programs, evaluation will be better served by the use of combined methods (i.e., quantitative and qualitative) rather than by use of any single method alone to capture behavioral change processes and outcomes. Subsequent chapters provide a detailed discussion of program evaluation and its various quantitative and qualitative methods.

To understand the role of evaluation in HIV/AIDS programs, it is essential to understand the environment in which such programs are presented and the target populations. Discussion of the characteristics of communities, the roles they can play in program development, implementation, and evaluation, and ways of assessing a community's educational and service delivery needs are presented in detail. Measurement issues, including types of assessment, data collection methods, and assessment of behavioral change and program effects are addressed, and examples from actual interventions are provided

Discussion of concepts pertaining to HIV/AIDS interventions sets the tone for the context of evaluation. This volume melds theory with practice, by illustrating strategies for evaluating HIV prevention programs through case examples of recognized leaders in the field. Interventions targeted to the individual and those targeted to communities or groups are distinguished. This somewhat artificial distinction relates to how an intervention is assessed rather than to its content, impact, and outcome. Clearly, the two levels are interrelated. We differentiate intervention designed to modify the knowledge, attitudes, and behaviors of a group from a broader, more comprehensive community-level intervention aimed at fostering an environment receptive to change. Changes in individual HIV risk and precautionary behaviors are facilitated by changes in community-level normative influences. What society defines as desirable social norms underpin the maintenance of individual- and community-level behavior change. Successful individual- and community-level preventive interventions result in behavioral change, which decreases the incidence and prevalence of HIV/AIDS.

Involving Communities in Evaluation

Program evaluation can provide a target community with information on the effectiveness of prevention efforts. While an evaluator may believe that a community should be receptive to anyone willing to provide resources to improve members' knowledge, satisfaction with their quality of life, and ultimately their health, this is not always the case. To develop realistic intervention goals and objectives and evaluation mechanisms, a community should be the focal point in identifying its own HIV/AIDS prevention needs. In the absence of community endorsement, external HIV/AIDS preventive interventions may be disconnected from the community.

Communities that are not sold on the appropriateness of an intervention may feel even less committed to its evaluation. Traditionally, the evaluation process has been viewed as useless and irrelevant because it does not bear tangible services. A community may perceive itself as the giver and the evaluator as an "outsider" who collects data and takes information from the community.

Community participation at every step of the program—assessing needs, developing partnerships, program planning, intervention implementation, and evaluation—is essential to get a community to embrace the need for evaluation. Members must see that evaluation will produce information that will benefit them.

This chapter focuses on how to become acquainted with a community, what an evaluation team needs to know to be accepted by that community, and how to assure that appropriate, targeted HIV/AIDS preventive interventions are delivered. The definition, diversity, and needs of a community and effective techniques for involving community members and fostering an evaluator's relationship with them are also addressed. The chapter concludes with recommendations on how evaluation results are disseminated in a final report.

EVALUATION'S BENEFITS FOR THE COMMUNITY

Communities and their institutions can benefit from program evaluation in four essential ways:

- First, active participation in the evaluation process provides a vehicle for mutual aid and community empowerment. Collaborating in an evaluation may decrease feelings of impotence in addressing HIV/AIDS in a community. Members may already feel powerless due to economic instability and lack of education.
- Second, a series of evaluations, both formative and summative, form a feedback loop with the target community. As described later in this volume, through

formative evaluation strategies, which involve ongoing dialogue with the community, appropriate program goals and objectives can and should be realized prior to program development and implementation. Summative evaluations enable educators to communicate back to the community intervention impact and outcome. This information keeps a community current on its members' HIV-related knowledge, adoption and maintenance of HIV risk-reduction behaviors, satisfaction with HIV prevention programs, and trends in the use of condoms, controlled substances, and incidence and prevalence of sexually transmitted diseases.

- Third, evaluation results may trigger changes in community norms. Examples of norms include condom use, HIV counseling and testing, seeking health care services (Mantell & DiVittis, 1990), or the perceived benefits of HIV-infected pregnant women taking zidovudine during pregnancy.
- Fourth, one result of evaluation and ongoing monitoring and dialogue with a community is to foster accountability to the community. This also establishes a direct link between individual community members and members of the evaluation team. In addition to information transfer, community members may expect evaluation researchers to assist them in obtaining funds for new programs.

DEFINITION AND DIVERSITY OF COMMUNITY

Community is most often defined as a geographic location or all the people who reside within a given area. It can also refer to a group of persons with an affiliation, such as a group of people living as a social unit, or a group with similar characteristics, e.g., interests, lifestyles, work, politics, risk factors, health conditions or disease, or culture. While it is easy to characterize a community in terms of its physical site, its demographics and spirit are more difficult to determine and understand. Characteristics that differentiate people in a community include age, gender, sexual orientation, ethnicity/race, income, education, occupation, religion, language, political affiliation, family group or affiliation, values and beliefs, health status, and service utilization. Classification as a community can emanate from personal identification by persons who have one or more characteristics in common or from labeling by others who view a group of persons as having common characteristics.

A person belongs to many overlapping communities concurrently. Depending on the time or situation, one or more of these community affiliations may be in the forefront, while others may be in the background. For example, 20- to 30-year-old gay men with AIDS living in New York City's Chelsea district reflect many dimensions of community, e.g., age, network affiliation, prevalence of various diseases, and physical location. In planning interventions with a community, note that self-identification is not static but can shift quickly depending on the issues at stake.

Demographic indicators can help an evaluator define a community and understand its needs. These data, however, do not explain the social, economic, political, and historical conditions surrounding the lives of community members. For example, despite the value of census data in describing community parameters, a number of important features are not captured, e.g., how many persons are undocumented and therefore uncounted, number of years particular immigrant groups have been living in the United States, and the cohesiveness of an immigrant community. Census data that are collected every 10 years in the United States do not provide timely identification of trends. In addition, relying on social and demographic indicators as the primary source of information about a community bypasses the opinions of its members and workers.

DEVELOPING A WORKING PARTNERSHIP WITH THE COMMUNITY

The Need for Community Participation

HIV/AIDS prevention goals and objectives, the strategies and interventions to achieve them, and the evaluation mechanisms for intervention implementation and impact must reflect the needs and culture of the target community. Community members and organizations have an understanding of and access to a community that is initially unavailable to the program planner and evaluator. Established community-based organizations and identified community leaders have a comprehension of the beliefs and practices of their constituents as well as a respect and believability among them. Years of experience have proven that, for change to occur, people must be directly involved in identifying their own needs, setting priorities, and planning programs. The evaluator, on the other hand, needs the community's confidence and support to gain access to: (1) information and other resources, (2) persons with a historical perspective, (3) informal power structures, and (4) communication channels for information dissemination.

Community participation is essential at the onset of planning for an intervention, during its implementation, and at each stage of evaluation and analysis. This includes the development of goals and objectives and research questions, selection of intervention strategies, interviewing, creation of curriculum and materials, input into the evaluation design, program implementation and maintenance, evaluation implementation, data analysis and interpretation, report writing, and dissemination of findings. For example, in a community-based research study in Uganda (Seeley, Kengeya-Kayondo, & Mulder, 1992), community members were initially recruited to map the study area and work as survey interviewers. These interviewers served as intermediaries between the local communities and research team, providing feedback on the communities' responses to the survey. Subsequently, some interviewers were redeployed to take a census, continue annual quantitative surveys, collect qualitative data, make home visits, and were eventually trained as counselors. They also provided consultation to the researchers regarding strategies for the census and health survey in each village.

Defining the problems to be addressed and the hypotheses to be tested, in particular, should be negotiated among various stakeholders, including the evaluator. If the community is not directly involved, evaluation can be perceived as something alien, imposed on the community by "outsiders" insensitive to existing cultural norms. This perception would most likely lead to ineffective program implementation and participation and to political handicapping of its evaluation. In addition, claims of a program's accountability may be meaningless if not accepted by those most closely involved.

To encourage commitment of scarce resources, community members need to understand the benefits of evaluation and the positive impact a combination of qualitative and quantitative data can have in securing funding for prevention programs and service delivery. Evaluators need to be aware of possible negative, undesirable, or unintended consequences that might be raised by community members. Additionally, because of their understanding of how the community works and the resources and barriers that impact behavior, community members can be immensely helpful in educating program planners and researchers about the community's needs and the best way to meet them. As such, the community representatives should not be merely figureheads that serve as "window dressing" for a steering committee, but *collaborators* with the program and evaluation team.

Building Consensus

Developing a collaborative relationship takes understanding, time, nurturing, and patience. Hatch, Moss, Saran, Presley-Cantrell, and Malloy (1993) believe collaborative research benefits the community through direct programs or services as well as through education of its members. Engaging community members as collaborators throughout the intervention and evaluation process will increase their commitment to the program and foster consensus planning and decision-making. In essence, this process forms a covenant between the program/evaluation team and the community. Here, each side has a clear set of expectations of the other. Provided that trust is not broken, this allows the team access to implement program goals and objectives and assess the degree to which they have been achieved.

Consensus within the community helps to insure that different segments of the population agree on the support they will lend, thus helping to curb opposition to the project. Once a partnership has been established, community organizations can be mobilized to support and reinforce community social norms that promote HIV-related prevention behaviors and programs (Braithwaite & Lythcott, 1989).

Further, by involving the community early in the process, the program/evaluation team is able to identify the work that has been done by the community and incorporate it into its prevention strategy. In an effort to understand why community-based organizations become involved in HIV/AIDS preventive interventions, Freudenberg, Lee, and Silver (1989) conducted a community-based study in New York City's Washington Heights. This predominantly Latino community has many established community-based organizations that address public health and social issues. Sixty percent of the 28 community organizations sampled had incorporated AIDS prevention activities, such as counseling programs for women and teens, community forums and health fairs, seminars for parents, and library-based programs and materials, into their programmatic repertoire. Developing links among existing community-based programs helped to assure HIV/AIDS interventions within a community already facing serious health and social problems. Programming areas that can facilitate the introduction and expansion of HIV/AIDS content include sexuality education, sexually transmitted disease (STD) prevention education, and drug-use education and treatment.

Acknowledging established roles in programming performs two functions: (1) an intervention team does not have to "reinvent the wheel" in the target community, and (2) by recognizing the preexisting efforts, the team further strengthens the coalition with the community. Otherwise, one risks being perceived as arrogant outsiders, interfering in a situation the community perceives it has well in hand.

Identifying the Community Infrastructure

Community institutions, such as the churches, industry, public and parochial schools, community boards, political leaders, social and sports clubs, and block associations, are key to promoting community-wide HIV prevention, intervention planning, and evaluation. These organizations and their members provide social networks, formal and informal power bases, and groups that define community norms and deviance.

Organizations' credibility within the community and their knowledge of the culture and values are essential to developing relevant HIV/AIDS prevention programs and evaluation strategies. These organizations, which maintain ongoing channels of communication, are the pipeline of the community. Many communities with large numbers of people infected or affected by HIV/AIDS are politically disenfranchised and besieged by extensive poverty, drug use, lack of affordable housing, and a dearth of adequate health care, problems that existed prior to the HIV epidemic. Most likely, there is an existing community infrastructure that has worked on these problems and could be tapped to coalesce around HIV.

Assuring Sensitivity to the Community

The community is not only the group to be served, but also those to whom AIDS prevention planners and evaluators are accountable. Besides being responsible to funders, boards, and institutions, evaluators are answerable to the community for the ethical integrity of the research, appropriate use of resources, and honest evaluation. To be successful, a program must reflect the culture and needs of the target community. Particular attention should be paid to determining whether the community has experienced a sense of exploitation and abandonment by research programs once the funding is over. This has often been the case among economically disadvantaged communities. Therefore, evaluators must have not only the professional skills to develop and complete an evaluation, but the awareness and sensitivity to work effectively with culturally diverse communities. In particular, the evaluator needs to know that the evaluation methods will be acceptable to the target population.

Formative evaluation techniques can help researchers feel the pulse and sensibilities of a community. By conducting formative evaluation of an HIV vaccine preparedness study, an evaluator will learn why community members are willing or unwilling to participate. To get community support for the evaluation, plans may need to be modified. Sometimes sensitivity to community needs has to take precedence over scientific merit and rigor of the evaluation.

Culture is an integrated system of learned customs, beliefs and values, knowledge, and skills that shape people's behavior patterns (Randall-David, 1994). Culture influences HIV-related beliefs (e.g., perceptions of HIV risk vulnerability, prejudice about drug users and homosexuals), use of condoms, pregnancy planning among HIV-infected women, ethnic and sexual identity, and gender roles.

Evaluators need to recognize the diversity in communities and not homogenize them into one group. For example, classifying "communities of color" (i.e., people who are diverse in their ethnicity and not white or of European descent) as a unitary group in an evaluation may obfuscate inter- and intragroup differences. Consider that Latinos differ from one another based on country of birth, racial background, socioeconomic status, geographic residence, number of years since immigration to the United States, legal status, degree of assimilation or acculturation, history of oppression, and other life experiences. Further, women who have sex with women include both women who have sex with women only and women who have sex with men and women. Drug users also are a diverse group, representing people from all ethnic backgrounds and many socio-economic classes. They differ from one another based on the type, duration, and frequency of their drug use. It is essential, therefore, for an evaluator to factor into the evaluation the effects of intra- and intergroup variability (Padilla & Salgado de Snyder, 1992).

An intervention and evaluation team should be sensitive to a community's historical experience with government-sponsored medical research, because this may affect community acceptance of intervention-based research. African Americans, in particular, may be reluctant to welcome educators and researchers into their communities, because historically this population has been abused, experimented upon, and exploited in medical research, as witnessed by the 1932 United States Public Health Service-funded Tuskegee study of untreated syphilitic black male sharecroppers (Thomas & Quinn, 1991; Gamble, 1993; Jones, 1993). This experiment serves as a potent reminder of the misguided governmental policies and underlies the belief of some African Americans that HIV is a racial attack on African Americans—a form of genocide (Thomas, 1991; Thomas & Morgan, 1991).

Distrust may also be a significant barrier to a community's acceptance of preventive HIV vaccines; this may ultimately lead to their not endorsing community members' participation in vaccine preparedness trials that include a behavioral risk-reduction intervention component.

Culturally competent HIV preventive interventions require the HIV prevention and evaluation team to be aware of their own beliefs, values, and culture (e.g., in relation to sexual practices, sexual orientation, drug use, persons from different ethnic groups) and how these factors impact intervention development, their work with the target population, and the evaluation process (Randall-David, 1994; Sue, Arredondo, & McDavis, 1992). Sometimes, cultural sensitivity to one group in a community may result in insensitivity to other groups. For example, promoting condom use as the primary means of sexual risk reduction may be acceptable to adolescents but unacceptable to parents and religious groups that endorse abstinence.

Even though understanding the members' cultural backgrounds may provide a guide to community attitudes, values, and behaviors, it is not a substitute for participation by community members and leaders.

Working with Community Coalitions

Gaining the support of community coalitions is one effective way for an evaluator to obtain the active participation of a community in program development, implementation, and evaluation. Coalitions are individuals or groups representing agencies and constituencies within the community who develop formal or informal working relationships based on issues of mutual interest.

Whether mandated or voluntary, coalitions are systems developed to maximize the use of dwindling resources. Their appeal lies in their ability to improve democratic representation, involve greater portions of the community in setting and implementing a community-identified agenda with goals and objectives, enhance organizational expertise, focus service coordination and efficiency, eliminate duplication of services, and develop advocacy and public policy. Factors identified as leading to successful coalitions include leadership and membership characteristics, members' perception of benefits and costs of participation, organizational climate and relations, as well as the decision-making process and skills for resolving conflict (Butterfoss, Goodman, & Wandersman, 1993). For example, the Request for Proposals for the HIV Vaccine Preparedness and Phase III Efficacy Trials by the National Institute on Allergy and Infectious Diseases called for assessing the extent of community support for preventive HIV vaccine trials. Researchers were required to form a community advisory board to focus on community concerns about the study protocols and educational and promotional materials.

The mandating of coalitions has become the norm for many funders, including federal, state, and city agencies. For some initiatives, The Robert Wood Johnson Foundation requires the existence of coalitions before application for funding. One successful candidate, the AIDS ARMS Network in Dallas, developed a coalition that has weekly meetings to address case management and service needs of persons with AIDS. In addition to sharing useful information with clients, these meetings are often support groups for providers who are members of the coalition (John Snow, Inc., 1993). In all cities receiving Ryan White funding, legislative regulations have required grant recipients to form planning councils to decide how funds will be used.

Understanding the ever-changing issues of a coalition is essential if one is evaluating a community intervention. Missions of a coalition may evolve, members and their power bases may change, and political environments in which they function may be altered.

Community-based organizations that serve HIV-infected clients need to be aware of and work with their service providers to assure that client needs are being met. Coalitions may be created from social service, religious, and public health-focused organizations, as well as those that are AIDS-specific. Members can be primary service providers, bureaucrats from public agencies such as social services, mental health, and housing, as well as advocates for persons with HIV/AIDS or those at risk. Organizations that have previously developed programs for drug users, women, adolescents, and minorities are often receptive to developing HIV networks that pool their resources for developing and evaluating preventive interventions.

Recently, in New York City, a coalition of consumers of HIV-related services was formed, called CHAIN (Community Health Advisory Information Network). Its function is to recruit a representative sample of New York City's HIV-positive community to identify its needs, service utilization patterns, and satisfaction with available services. A total of 698 consumers of HIV-related services in the five boroughs of New York were randomly selected from the rolls of community-based AIDS service organizations (ASOs), clinics, hospitals, and other related institutions. Interviews with members of this sample were conducted to identify service needs (including unmet needs), overall health, and social service utilization, as well as satisfaction with the service system. Baseline data were collected on the initial sample, and follow-up interviews have been completed on 300, in order to gauge changes over time. Information is being disseminated to the HIV planning council, under the auspices of the New York City mayor's office. The planning council is charged with the task of distributing the city's HIV Ryan White CARE Act allotment. Work groups of the council are preparing an implementation plan for fiscal year 1996. The information provided by CHAIN is being factored into that implementation plan and preparation of a 3-year strategic plan for New York City. In addition, information obtained from CHAIN will be shared with the service organizations from which the sample was drawn. This will enable the ASOs and other HIV service providers to incorporate consumer input into their programs, and it will provide information as to how area consumers view the degree to which their needs are met (D. Abramson, personal communication).

The Adolescent AIDS Network in New York City, composed of more than 100 organizations, focuses on adolescent health issues, provides consultation and updates on city and state policies, shares curricula with member agencies, and develops political strategies to maintain programs and their funding.

Development and maintenance of coalitions or interorganizational networks may also pose some drawbacks. These include a lack of trust based on past funding competition among the organizations, lack of a policy document and cooperative procedures, unclear roles and responsibilities, different organizational philosophies, exclusion of particular groups, insufficient funding, lack of active communication channels, difficulty in reaching a consensus, and competing interests of the individual organization and the network.

The successes and problems encountered in creating and maintaining an AIDS network are illustrated in the case study of the National AIDS Community Action Network in Chile described below (Anderson, Frasca, & Gauthier, 1995).

Case Study of the Chilean National AIDS Community Action Network

The History

In 1991, a variety of community religious, women's, gay, and human rights groups working in HIV/AIDS in Chile recognized the need to empower organizations and their clients by sharing information, educational strategies, and resources. Following the First National Ecumenical Pastoral Conference on AIDS and two seminars to discuss the need for expanded HIV prevention and service provision, the AIDS Community Action Network (ACAN) was established.

Contract of Participation

Different motivations for joining the network led to disproportionate participation. While some organizations joined to further their own agendas, others believed that the network was a way to develop an integrated AIDS prevention plan that could influence governmental policies and actions. To codify participants' expectations, a contract was developed that requested: (1) consistent participation in monthly meetings; (2) payment of monthly dues based on a sliding scale; (3) adherence to ACAN's Declaration of Principles; and (4) commitment to complete promised tasks.

Competing Needs

Organizational tasks meant abandoning some responsibilities in their own non-governmental organization. There was a problem with recognition of ACAN's work but not the individual members. This caused particular tension because the extra work competed with work essential to funders and clients. With long-term involvement, the competition of time requirements between the individual organization and ACAN, as well as the benefits of the work, was something participants needed to be aware of.

Leadership

The lack of a designated leader was identified as a potential problem. While the organization had no full-time staff or a process for delegating responsibility, the development of structures was also perceived as problematic. There was a concern that the network would evolve into another superumbrella organization rather than a democratic social movement composed of many groups and leaders. Employment of a part-time secretary and establishment of a separate office helped to provide some structure for administrative duties. All other activities were performed by volunteers.

Activism

Homosexual behavior is unlawful in Chile. However, gay groups were instrumental in developing AIDS awareness and programming, and more recently they became politically active and confrontational in advocating for gay rights. This agenda has often been in opposition to ACAN's educational emphasis on the topics of homosexuality and AIDS. ACAN is in a continuing dialogue with the gay community to address sexual rights in the broader context of human rights. Community-based organizations are not autonomous; the government funds many of their current programs. Any political activity on the part of this network that opposes government policy puts individual organizations' funding in jeopardy. Therefore, network members need to develop strategies to retain their independence, while working effectively with the government.

Funding

Network building has been stressed as a way to promote cost-beneficial HIV/AIDS interventions, collectively organized activities, and community development of policy.

Yet, international funders have neglected to develop policies that recognize and reward such networks with separate funding streams or consultation roles for funding decisions about their individual members.

Successes

Following some initial trial and error during the establishment of the network structure, ACAN evolved into a network of 24 organizations that meet monthly. A three-person committee was elected to coordinate the network, with assistance from a special events commission. Grant-funded activities have included World AIDS Day activities, a candlelight memorial, and a workshop that helped to establish a municipally funded AIDS network in Santiago.

Network problems such as those identified in the above case example can be resolved with effort. To assist in organizing a network and its goals and objectives, a series of documents should be drafted, including a description of membership criteria, a mission statement, and flowsheets or workplans to evaluate progress and success. Daily administration can be facilitated by a part-time employee housed in a separate network office or the office of one of the community-based organizations. There is a need to recognize the pull of commitments between the network and the individual organizations. Actual shared work experience, such as developing a workshop or conference, helps to build trust and facilitate learning among network members. Monetary resources and time resources are usually limited in community-based organizations. To facilitate communication among members, monthly meetings can be augmented by phone contact and use of the Internet. External and internal changes must be constantly addressed to maintain a successful HIV coalition.

Coalitions and Behavioral Change

Coalitions can be the driving force for community-level behavioral change. Assessment methods for evaluating community changes due to coalition activities have not yet been fully developed or reported in the literature (McElroy, Kegler, Steckler, Burdine, & Wisotzky, 1994). For example, if an evaluator wants to know whether a community has mobilized successfully to embrace HIV risk reduction, the effectiveness of planning activities and outcomes could be assessed by such indicators as formation of by-laws, identification of new objectives, the formation of new community groups to work on HIV prevention, and coalition members' satisfaction with the planning process and outcomes. In addition, the ability of a coalition to secure funds for HIV prevention programs and their evaluation is another potential indicator of its planning success.

An Evaluation Model Involving the Community

Figure 2.1 presents a model of comprehensive evaluation in the context of working with, rather than around, the target community (Mantell & DiVittis, 1990). A series of goals and objectives, which formulate the framework of an HIV preventive intervention, flow from the needs assessment. This in turn focuses the evaluation strategy (i.e., the

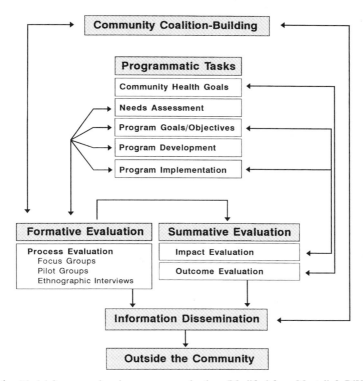

Figure 2.1.   Model for comprehensive program evaluation. (Modified from Mantell & DiVittis, 1990.)

degree to which the program has met the identified needs). A community's collective needs require a program to address the ultimate goal of HIV prevention: to reduce the incidence of HIV infection in the community. A program that will best meet this long-term health goal can then be developed.

The model is predicated on the value of communication among the community, program developers, and the evaluator. This continuous feedback loop keeps the evaluator abreast of changes in the community, while providing the community with information on the impact the intervention is having on its constituents. Information is further disseminated outside the loop to other health educators, social scientists, and communities.

PRESENTING RESULTS OF AN EVALUATION TO A COMMUNITY OF COMMUNITY-BASED ORGANIZATIONS

After a program evaluation has been completed, an AIDS service organization often needs to present findings to its board, funders, decision-makers, or various community groups. Planning for analysis should be done by the evaluator in conjunction with the community-based organization (CBO) program staff and the community. The insights of the community will facilitate the accurate interpretation of results.

The first issue to address is how program questions have been answered. Conclusions are of two types: (1) those that are descriptive, and (2) those that present evidence of cause-and-effect relationships (Wendt, 1965). To establish cause and effect, an evaluator would have to be able to say that his or her intervention, rather than some other factor, was responsible for the program effect. The evaluator and research staff should discuss how evaluation findings will be organized and presented. Several versions may be needed to make the report relevant to different audiences; content should be of interest to the intended audience and strengthen their understanding. A complete technical report with detailed description of the data collection methods and procedures, an executive summary, and an abbreviated summary for distribution to practitioners, other agencies, and community groups will be required.

The report should present a statement of the problem: why a particular program needed to be evaluated. Methods used in the evaluation should be detailed. Another section should be devoted to program impact. Results should be presented in a straightforward fashion; the evaluator can then offer interpretations of these findings and their implications for the future. It must be kept in mind that there is the potential for sensitive findings. Strategies for reporting them should consider the community for whom the intervention was designed.

Though frequently reticent or discouraged by CBO management, an evaluator should present negative or "no differences" results and account for why this might have occurred. This kind of discussion provides a starting point for the next program, so that a "weak" program can be strengthened and additional people are not exposed to an ineffective intervention. Further, the community has a right and need to know the full range of the components of the intervention and their differential impact. This will help to highlight the breadth of the efforts put forth and degree to which they succeeded.

One way in which to present findings is to organize them according to the questions addressed by the evaluation. Tables and graphs should be clearly presented and the accompanying narrative should explain the data. The use of subheadings throughout the report can enhance its readability. When evaluation is utilization-focused, the final report may only be the culmination of a participatory process between the evaluator, health educator, and decision-makers (Patton, 1978). Suggested components of a final evaluation report are presented in Table 2.1.

DISSEMINATION OF THE RESULTS

Evaluators have a responsibility to ensure that, in addition to agency administration, program evaluation findings are disseminated to community members. Exchange and information between an evaluator and the target population should be bidirectional. All too often, this step in the feedback loop process is neglected, and communities feel that they have been taken advantage of or used by the evaluation team and/or the CBO. Dissemination of study results, however, should be negotiated with the CBO and larger community, preferably before the evaluation begins. This is all the more important if

GOALS AND OBJECTIVES: THE KEY TO EVALUATION

In general, evaluation of an HIV/AIDS preventive intervention, like the program itself, is focused and goal-driven. The overall goals and objectives of a program formulate the expected outcome of the evaluation itself.

A goal refers to the overall change in the community-at-large that the program developers and the evaluators expect to see, i.e., the intended consequences of the intervention. It is a general statement, not immediately measurable. An example of a goal of an HIV preventive intervention would be to foster risk reduction.

Objectives are the intermediate steps required to achieve intervention goals. An objective refers to the measurable or observable impact of the program on its participants or on another program "ingredient," e.g., "to develop five educational modules covering topics A, B, and C." This is similar to the effect expected by a scientist on the subjects of his or her experiment. To increase condom use by 15% among homeless men, one program objective might be to increase their access to condoms by distributing condoms through street-based outreach. Objectives are used to formulate the evaluation questions to be studied. The goals and objectives of an evaluation should be described in simple, straightforward terms and should be realistic and time-specific.

As a general guide, we can look to the five criteria, suggested by Leviton and Valdiserri (1990), to determine the benefits of HIV/AIDS prevention programs, especially the extent to which new HIV infections decline in at-risk populations as a result of participation. These include the probability that an at-risk individual will:

- be identified
- be recruited into the program
- be provided with AIDS prevention education
- reduce or eliminate risky behaviors
- reduce his or her personal risk for HIV infection

This strategy provides a basic framework that will enable the evaluator to determine goals and objectives that are participant-centered and include all phases of program evaluation.

One goal of a preventive intervention might be that the community will adopt safer sex practices or that HIV infection rates will be reduced in the target population. These goals capture the overall intent of the prevention program but are not readily measurable and do not guide program implementation. Rather, they capture the overall outcome of the program.

Objectives that quantify each of these general goals will enable the evaluator to provide feedback on the success of the process of the program (e.g., recruitment techniques), as well as the impact the program had on participant behavior (e.g., the number of participants who adopted safer sex practices after program participation).

In either case, the goals and objectives of the evaluation are part of the overall prevention strategy. Program effectiveness is related to the overall intervention strategy and the care and thought that went into its design. In other words, you can only evaluate what you have got. A programmer who did not design a prevention program to increase safer sex negotiation skills should not be surprised if, upon evaluation, the program was found to be ineffective in increasing the participants' skills.

THE RESEARCH QUESTIONS: WHAT ARE WE TRYING TO LEARN?

Essentially, all HIV prevention specialists are trying to find an evaluation strategy that answers the same question: Did the program work? The only problem with such a question is that, as stated, it is unanswerable. Two essential questions are embedded in the simple query, "did it work"? First, what is "it"? Second, what does "work" mean? The type of questions needed are those that can be answered empirically as well as meaningfully.

One of the major issues confronting AIDS organizations is determining what research questions to ask. Organizations may need an evaluator's assistance in framing the research questions. All too often, questions are posed inarticulately or in vague terms. As noted by Patton (1978), the framing of the research questions should be an interactive process between the evaluator and the CBO. Discussion is needed so that the AIDS organization's staff can agree on the research questions, goals, and objectives of the evaluation. The evaluator can be useful in articulating and clarifying the issues of interest, intent of the evaluation, and developing the criteria to be evaluated.

Formulating the research questions are as important as the technical aspects of the evaluation. Although this could entail a lengthy process, such focus may yield a significant payoff in terms of useful results to both the agency and the evaluator. Evaluation can become more credible if the CBO staff participates in determining the questions to be answered by the evaluation.

Also, in focusing the research questions, the AIDS organization and evaluator should explicitly realize what questions will not be answered by the evaluation. Understanding the limitations of an evaluation strategy is essential for both parties. Sometimes an evaluator can suggest alternative ways of defining a problem, helping the CBO staff understand substantive and methodological issues (Berk & Rossi, 1990).

The evaluator needs to be assured at the outset that he or she is answering the questions the organization really wants to know. This avoids wasting resources on answering the wrong questions and prevents conflict or mistaken expectations. In developing an evaluation protocol, the evaluator should know how the evaluation will be used—how it will inform program operations and policy.

The research questions will also drive the choice of study design, data collection methods, and assessment procedures to be used in the evaluation. Lack of clarity in questions can create confusion about the overall measurement approach. However, the interests of the evaluators and program developers will often be curtailed by the fiscal limitations of the funders and organizations for whom the evaluation is being conducted. In general, the availability of staff, money, and other organizational support resources will determine how the evaluation will be implemented.

TYPES OF PROGRAM EVALUATION

Program evaluation is not an exact science. It is important for the reader to keep in mind that a program evaluation can be executed in a number of ways, the complexity of which is driven by the objectives of the organization, the questions that need to be answered, and the resources available to implement the evaluation. We focus on evaluations that are process-oriented and summative in this section.

Process Evaluation

Process evaluation involves a variety of techniques that enable the evaluator to assess the quality of an HIV prevention program. Information collected includes an assessment of the efficiency of program execution, replicability, monitoring, quality control, and content while the program is operating, utilization of the program, perceived program effectiveness, and participant satisfaction.

Diverse methods of assessment are used in process evaluation. Both qualitative and quantitative data collection are included. Qualitative data refer to information that is described in word rather than numeric format. A detailed discussion of qualitative methods is presented in Chapter 7. Qualitative data include information collected from open-ended items on questionnaires and unstructured interviews where the respondent is asked about his or her feelings, concerns, and issues associated with HIV. Information gathered in an open-ended interview, such as a focus group, for the purposes of identifying the needs of a community, is another example of qualitative data.

Quantitative data are numeric in nature. Here, items are structured and assigned a metric prior to data collection. The information gathered includes such things as counting (e.g., How much time was spent discussing safer sex in a workshop? How many intervention sessions did a participant attend? What is the rate of participant attrition over the course of an intervention? How many participants were referred for HIV counseling and testing?) and responses to surveys designed to assess variables of interest (e.g., On a scale of 1 to 10, where 1 represents completely dissatisfied and 10 represents completely satisfied, rate your satisfaction with the workshop and/or facilitator). Both are valuable and applicable to process evaluation. Table 3.1 presents a summary of some of the advantages and disadvantages of qualitative and quantitative approaches.

When information is collected to select the most effective intervention tools or enhance or improve the program, it is referred to as a *formative evaluation*. When data are collected to monitor how the program has been conducted, it is referred to as *implementation evaluation* or *program monitoring*.

Formative Evaluation

Formative evaluation focuses on the collection of process-oriented information with the purpose of improving the program. Formative evaluation begins with the creation of the program, in the identification of the community's needs, through its implementation. Through feedback via needs assessment surveys, interviews with key informants and "gatekeepers," pretests, focus groups, monitoring surveys, and observations, an evaluator is able to propose constructive changes in both the program development and implementation stages. It is often a first step in the evaluation process—a discovery and exploration phase.

One of the initial phases of the formative evaluation is the needs assessment. This process enables the program staff to determine the fit between the program and the needs

Table 3.1. Advantages and Disadvantages
of Quantitative and Qualitative Data Collection Methods

Quantitative	Qualitative
Advantages	
Both inductive and deductive approach	Inductive approach
Reliability and validity of data assessed through standard analytic techniques	Allows for greater interpersonal contact between interviewer and respondents
Provides standardized assessment	Permits in-depth probing of knowledge, attitudes, and behaviors
Describes variation in a population's characteristics	Clarifies process and implementation problems
Measures program effects	Effective means for discussing sensitive issues (e.g., sexual behavior and drug use)
Provides summary or aggregate measures	
Structured data collection	Provides important contextual data that can amplify meaning of quantitative findings
	Sheds light on the developmental processes and meanings from the respondent's perspective
	Generates new hypotheses; effective for research and study development
Limitations	
Requires larger samples than qualitative evaluation studies	Weaker internal validity than quantitative findings
	Limited generalizability of findings
Lacks detailed information about contextual background of attitudes and behaviors	With focus group methods, some group members may not participate in discussion; individual variation may be obscured
	Tends to be more labor-intensive and can be expensive, depending on number of staff, length of time in field, and complexity of coding scheme and data analysis

of the target population. In addition to identifying the needs of a given group, a needs assessment can also address the most appropriate way to implement the program or, beyond that, what type of program is needed. Some of the techniques used in a needs assessment are questionnaires, interviews, and focus groups (see Chapter 4, for a more detailed discussion on needs assessment).

Unlike other forms of evaluation, formative evaluation provides a feedback loop that begins at the onset of program development, the primary task of which is to define process-oriented questions and create data collection techniques to enhance or improve the program over time. Key to the successful formative evaluation is the time frame for altering the intervention. Here, the information actually can be used to modify or improve the program. For example, the initial implementation of an HIV/AIDS risk-reduction program at Gay Men's Health Crisis (GMHC) in New York City used a six-session, small-group experience to modify sexual behavior among gay and bisexual men. The program used small-group exercises, role plays, games, group discussion, and support to incorporate didactic information. Feedback from debriefings with the facilitators and participant satisfaction surveys indicated that a four-session workshop would be a more acceptable means of presenting the information. Participants and facilitators indicated that a six-session workshop entailed too much commitment and that the information could be imparted in fewer sessions. There was a 2-month period between initial program implementation and its follow-up. During this period, program developers modified the intervention to reduce it to four sessions, make it more focused, and incorporate more experiential learning exercises (Mantell & DiVittis, 1989). Hence, it is critical to build in time for modifying the intervention based on the formative evaluation's findings.

A second purpose of formative evaluation is to determine the appropriateness and effectiveness of intervention tools (Miller & Cassel, in press). When applied prior to program implementation, it can save the organization time and money as well as spare the participants exposure to inappropriate interventions. In one example, GMHC's Internal Evaluation Unit performed a formative evaluation on the acceptability of two forms of a brochure. The first form was designed to appeal to an audience with a low reading level. Rather than being appealing, the brochure was seen as condescending to the people it was aimed to reach. The evaluation saved the agency thousands of dollars and spared the target audience from an inappropriate intervention (Miller & Cassel, in press).

Implementation Evaluation

Process evaluation of an HIV preventive intervention examines the implementation of a program. Here, implementation evaluation or program monitoring assesses what and how well the original intervention plan was implemented and documents those changes needed to insure proper replication. Implementation evaluation does not determine how effective a program is. It can lead, however, to recommendations about quality control to program developers.

Implementation evaluation also is aimed at monitoring the management of the program as well as service delivery. Was the intervention implemented as intended? Is the implementation schedule replicable? This applies to the process of implementation as well as the content to be implemented. For example, if the intervention plan called for half of a 60-minute session to be spent on a discussion of sexual risk-reduction practices and the other half on drug-related risk-reduction practices, the following process evaluation questions would need to be answered:

- Were 30 minutes allotted to each topic?
- Was the time allotted adequate for the topics covered?
- What changes in format are necessary to better meet the goals and objectives of this session?

These program implementation checks can be conducted with the use of trained observers. An observer can determine whether there was consistency in terms of information presented and in the format of the intervention's implementation. Specifically, whether a group facilitator adhered to the program's agenda, covered material in the scheduled time, and the extent of interaction between the facilitator and group members (e.g., the number of times the facilitator talked; the number of times group members talked; facilitators' interpersonal sensitivity) can be assessed. Participant ratings can also be used to monitor quality control, either through self-administered questionnaires or more in-depth interviews with a sample of participants. The questions in Table 3.2 were designed for a process evaluation of an AIDS education program implemented in gay bars over a 1-year period.

To determine the answers to the above questions, systematic data collection tools are required. One example of such a tool is called the program evaluation milestone (PEM) chart, as shown in Table 3.3. The PEM format, similar to a program evaluation and review technique (PERT) chart, enables the program developer, health educator, or evaluator to identify the series of tasks involved in the development of the prevention program and to monitor the progress of each activity over time. In this example, the PEM chart is used as an evaluation tool in the quarterly monitoring of an AIDS prevention intervention. As a management tool, the PEM provides an estimation of program "costs." It enables people who are running the program to keep tabs on the amount of time required for each aspect of the program. It also provides others with a tested and more realistic time frame to run the same program in other locations.

Proper data collection techniques can assist in determining the success of a program. One technique used in the GMHC Research Program was a facilitator summary sheet. Program facilitators were carefully trained in how to gather requisite information for a given session. Data collection on the process of implementation helped monitor the amount of variation in program delivery and resulted in uniformity of reporting. After each session, program facilitators were contacted by the research program staff to review what happened during the session.

Table 3.4 gives an example of a facilitator session summary sheet used for Project HEART, an AIDS prevention program for residents in a drug-free therapeutic community (TC). Prior to conducting a session, summary sheets were prepared for each facilitator. The information gathered included key identifiers (i.e., facilitator's name and phone number, site identifier number, and time of session) and the interviewer's impressions. The interview with the group facilitator addressed basic questions such as, "Did

---

Table 3.2.   Process Measures for an AIDS Education Program in Gay Bars[a]

- Were all the intervention deadlines met?
- Were the numbers of targeted people reached?
- How were group facilitators selected?
- How was the sample of participants selected?
- Were the facilitators on time?
- Were the facilitators skilled in leading the group discussions?
- Did the intervention outline represent a reasonable match to the participants encountered?
- Is the program replicable in its current format?
- How many staff and volunteers were required to conduct this program?
- What were the sociodemographic characteristics of participants?
- Was the intervention's setting accessible and conducive to participants?
- What did the participants see as the strengths of the on-site gay bar program?
- What were the perceived weaknesses of the on-site gay bar program; what would the participants have changed?

[a]From Mantell et al. (1989a).

Table 3.3. Program Evaluation Milestones
for an AIDS Preventive Intervention in Gay Bars[a]

Program	Task	Q_1	Q_2	Q_3	Q_4[b]
Bar program	Questionnaire development	△	•		
	Protocol finalized	△	•		
	Publicity design	△	•		
	External review		•		
	Site determination	△	△	•	
	Media release (ads, etc.)			•	
	Facilitator training			•	
	Pretest			•	
	Interventions			•	
	Posttest			•	
	Coding of data			△	•
	On-site observation		△	•	
	Follow-up				•
	Data analysis			△	•
	Final report	△	△	△	•

[a]From Mantell *et al.* (1989a).
[b]Q_1 to Q_4, quarter of the year, first through fourth; △, work in progress; •, work completed.

the session begin on time?" "What topics were covered?" "Was the time allotted for each exercise sufficient?" This feedback from facilitators across sessions provided the research program staff with information necessary to determine format changes over the different sessions. Further, after completion of the program, all facilitators were invited to meet with the research program staff to share issues that arose in the implementation of Project HEART. This enabled the evaluators to assess the consistency of intervention implementation. By this we mean: Were all participants exposed to the same intervention? Were the components of the intervention equally weighted across presentations? Was there a difference in attendance rates by session? If so, what caused these differences?

Some of this information was also shared with administrators and frontline coun-

Table 3.4. Facilitator Session Summary Sheet

Project HEART facilitator contact sheet

Facilitator name: Miguel Parades[a]	Group number: 4
Day phone: 555-6872	
Meeting day/time: Tuesday, 7:30–9:30	Location: TC #1

Staff contact with facilitator

Date	Time	Session	Comments
6/4/88	3:00	5	The facilitator reported some resistance on the part of the men to discuss loss of erection during condom use in front of the women in the group.

[a]Not facilitator's real name.

selors at the TC. For example, one of the issues that emerged in group discussions with facilitators was that residents believed that the Project HEART group was the only venue within the TC to discuss AIDS. This was due to a misunderstanding of the confidentiality rule—"What is said in this room, stays in this room." Hence, the participants did not perceive that they had a forum for discussing AIDS-related concerns in their daily TC life. This problem was brought to the attention of TC program and administrative staff, who along with research program staff, identified the need to integrate future AIDS programs into TC residents' daily living activities. Such integration should, optimally, open residents to multiple venues of AIDS information, create a community-centered power base for dealing with such issues, and eliminate the need to internalize their feelings about AIDS.

In process evaluation, it is helpful to obtain as much information from as many sources as possible. This enables the AIDS evaluator to assess the congruence among what was proposed (program), what was presented (facilitator), and what was received (participant). Hence, gathering of participant data is the third vital application of process evaluation. This can be achieved by site visits that entail observation and taking notes about the process of a session. For example, in a program to train a group of low-income women as AIDS educators and counselors, staff might observe training sessions to assess whether the training curriculum addresses the type of problems that arise in an HIV counseling session with women and whether the counselors are adequately prepared to deliver needed AIDS information. Additionally, through observation, staff can evaluate whether trainees have the requisite skills to deliver the educational message in compliance with the counselor-training protocol.

These evaluation techniques could well be problematic on two levels. First, this is a labor-intensive procedure that requires training staff to observe and record process, getting them to the site, and providing them with time to write the report. On a second, and equally important level, group members often will need to have developed mutual trust among themselves before agreeing to have an observer present. The presence of an outsider may be intrusive and could, in effect, interfere with the group bonding process and accomplishment of program objectives. In addition, if one group refuses to have an observer present, information from the observation cannot be gathered. This could distort the evaluator's overall understanding of how well the groups were functioning. These missing data result in a more limited view of how much variation there was among the groups and, therefore, the evaluator's ability to determine the degree to which intervention content was consistently presented across groups.

Another means of obtaining information about the way a program was run is to ask participants directly for their impressions in a questionnaire. Table 3.5 provides an example of selected questions used to evaluate participants' reactions to Project HEART. The questionnaire has two functions. First, it elicits participants' impressions regarding the way the program was implemented. For example, by directly asking participants about their satisfaction with session length and group size, AIDS educators can make informed decisions regarding the viability of replicating the program with the same session length and group size. Second, information gathered from the participants can be used to validate the impressions gathered from facilitators. It provides a form of checks and balances between the two data sources.

the number of participants attending and length of session, often with a precoded checklist. The same collection technique is qualitative when the observer is writing out his or her impressions of the group process.

Impact measures are frequently limited to assessment of knowledge and attitudinal measures and sometimes behavioral intentions. When long-term follow-up of participants cannot be conducted (for example, when their involvement in the program is anonymous, or it would be difficult to gain access to them at an agency or in their homes), assessment of short-term program outcomes may be the most viable option. Table 3.7 presents impact indicators assessing women's self-protective behavior from AIDSCAP's Women's Initiative (AWI) (Ankrah, 1996b) and the World Health Organization's Global Programme on AIDS. Although these measures have been widely used, Ankrah and the AWI (1996a) recognize that a woman's biological and behavioral processes require gender-specific and culturally sensitive measures of prevention impact. For example, they suggest that since STDs in women are often asymptomatic, impact measures of tertiary prevention of STDs are inadequate. Rather, inclusion of measures of secondary prevention behavior (e.g., increased number of STD screenings) will provide a more complete measure of women's self-protective behavior. In addition, the bottom-line approach to impact evaluation ignores vital internal processes (e.g., thinking about the need to adopt the behaviors) related to program success. In addition to impact on the individual, AWI calls for the need to include outcome measures, such as community-level normative change.

The expected amount of change necessary to declare a program successful should be specified. This will provide concrete and measurable indication of program success. Examples 3.1 and 3.2 illustrate measurement of short-term program outcomes.

Another study assessed the impact of an AIDS education comic on knowledge, attitudes, and behavioral intentions of 14-year-old English secondary school students, as shown in Example 3.2. Thus, evaluation of this controlled school education trial demonstrated the comic's short-term impact of improving AIDS-related knowledge levels. Impact evaluation of an intervention can consist of participant ratings as well as assessment of participants' self-reported changes in targeted results. An example of participant-rated items administered as part of a 6- and 12-month postintervention interview with women enrolled in methadone treatment to assess program impact is presented Table 3.8.

A range of relevant behaviors within the KAB domains should be analyzed simultaneously, using multivariate statistical methods (e.g., multiple regression), to

Table 3.7.   Indicators to Measure Impact of an AIDS Intervention in Increasing Women's Ability for Self-Protection[a]

- Increase in the proportion of women who report ever using a male or female condom
- Increase in the proportion of women who perceive they might be infected with HIV
- Increase in the proportion of women who report having made changes in sexual behavior to avoid HIV transmission
- Increase in the percentage of women who have the skills to negotiate use of the male or female condom
- Percentage of women's groups and community leaders who recognize the threat of HIV infection to women and men

[a]From Ankrah (1996b), with permission.

Example 3.1. Impact Evaluation

Evaluation Strategy

The impact of a soap opera videotape dealing with knowledge about the need for condoms, attitudes toward condom use, and the redemption of condom coupons on STD patients at Boston City Hospital was evaluated. The videotape presented condom use as a way of preventing AIDS and other STDs, and depicted its use as sexually appealing and socially acceptable.

While waiting for lab results, STD patients were solicited for study participation. Consenting subjects were randomly assigned to an intervention or a control group. Both intervention and control subjects were asked questions about their sociodemographic background, STD history, number of sexual partners in the past month, and their frequency of condom use. Following the interview, intervention subjects were shown the soap opera videotape.

Subjects then completed a checklist to assess whether they could recall the video's main points. Knowledge of STDs and proper condom use and strategies to persuade partners to use condoms were assessed in both intervention and control groups.

Results

Subjects who saw the videotape scored higher on the knowledge scale, were more favorably disposed to using condoms, and cited more strategies to persuade their partners to use condoms than did control subjects. The videotape proved to be most effective in terms of knowledge change for subjects with less formal education, for those who had never used condoms, and for those with only one sexual partner in the month prior to study participation. With respect to attitudes about condom use, the intervention was most effective for subjects with less formal schooling and those who were foreign-born.

(SOURCE: Solomon & DeJong, 1989.)

---

obtain a fuller picture of HIV risk-reduction (Leviton & Valdiserri, 1990). Such an analysis permits an examination of the interplay between variables and the roles they play in accounting for behavior change.

Data collection strategies are limited in that researchers generally do not have the opportunity to observe intimate sexual behaviors and needle sharing. Researchers have had to rely on subjects' self-reports. Although techniques to evaluate the reliability (i.e., consistency of measurement) and validity (accuracy of tool to measure what it purports to measure) of self-reported behaviors do exist, often AIDS researchers have not taken the additional step of checking the accuracy of their data (or at least do not report such psychometric analyses—assessing the integrity of measurement instruments—in the literature). The inclusion of social desirability scales (measures of the likelihood that the respondent is presenting self in a positive light) provides a check for the validity of self-reported health, sexual, and drug-related behaviors (quantitative measurement issues are discussed in Chapter 6).

It is important to note that the development of these measures is a science in and of

---

Example 3.2. Impact Evaluation

Evaluation Strategy

As a part of a controlled trial, an experimental group of 122 English secondary school students received the AIDS education comic and were matched—by geographic location, school size, and type and socioeconomic composition of catchment area—with a control group of 172 students who did not receive the comic. All students completed a questionnaire prior to the intervention and again, 2 weeks later.

Results

The group who had read and discussed the comic possessed a significantly higher level of knowledge (protective effects of condoms in reducing the risk of HIV transmission; sharing needles increases the risk of HIV infection; having only one sexual partner can reduce the risk of HIV transmission) at posttesting than those students who had not read the comic. There were, however, few statistically significant differences in group attitudes and behavioral intentions.

(SOURCE: Gillies & Stork, 1988.)

---

itself. The CBO will rarely have the staff with the expertise to develop questionnaires, surveys, and interview protocols. It is recommended that whenever possible, organizations utilize preexisting measures reported in the literature. In any event, documenting the reliability of the instrument on your chosen sample is a recommended practice (see Chapter 6).

If available, medical record data can be used to document the presence or absence of STDs, such as gonorrhea, chancroid, and syphilis, and hence can serve as an indicator of sexual behavioral change. In the absence of biological markers, changes in other similar variables (proxies) are used as indirect measures by which to draw inferences about program effectiveness. For example, simulated role plays about sexual and drug-related risk-reduction can be used as proxy (substitute) measures to evaluate the effectiveness of a skills training program.

In assessing program impact, evaluators also need to decide whether behavioral change will be examined on an item-by-item basis, that is, changes associated with a specific practice over time or in relation to a group of practices, for example, sexual practices that promote semen exchange. While it may be easier to interpret changes in individual practices, the grouping or scaling of related practices results in greater statistical power or sensitivity to the presence of program effects, but at the expense of exacting some precision (Connell *et al.*, 1988). For example, if you were assessing the impact of the program on the increase of alternative practices to sexual intercourse (e.g., body massage, playing with partner's nipples, and dry humping), an average of these individual behaviors would be more sensitive to statistically significant change, since the average reduces background noise (measurement error). However, precision in terms of which behaviors were most subject to change as a function of the intervention is lost. Similarly, when combining practices into a scale or summary measure, it is important

Table 3.8. Selected Participant Ratings
of an Intervention to Assess Short-Term Program Impact[a]

Now we would like to ask you a few questions about the health classes (sessions) you attended.

Q218. How many sessions of Project HOPE did you attend?   ____

#SESION6 __/__/

Q219. How much *new* information did the classes give you in the areas of _____ ?

	None	Little	Some	A lot
Pregnancy planning/birth control	0	1	2	3
BCINF6 __/__/				
VD	0	1	2	3
VDINF6 __/__/				
Safer sex	0	1	2	3
SAFESX6 __/__/				
Safer needle use	0	1	2	3
NEELDEU6 __/__/				
HIV/AIDS	0	1	2	3
HIVINF6 __/__/				
How to talk with partner about sex	0	1	2	3
PARTALK6 __/__/				
Reproductive/sexual organs	0	1	2	3
HUMBODY6 __/__/				

Q222. Have you discussed what you learned   ____ 01. No   ____ 02. Yes
about AIDS, safe sex, and birth
control with your partner?

TOLDPRT6 __/__/

Q223. Has your partner's behavior changed?   ____ 01. No   ____ 02. Yes

If Yes, tell me exactly how? _____

CHNGHOW6 __/__/

SHOW CARD 16

Q227. Finally, please tell me anything you think we ought to know about this interview and/or HIV/AIDS.

_____

FEELSA6 __/__/

_____

FEELSB6 __/__/

_____

FEELSC6 __/__/

[a]From Lanza, Hernandez, & Mantell (1991).

that the practices be highly related. For example, combining different forms of sexual intercourse (anal, vaginal, and oral) actually reduces the specificity of your measurement. The reason is that perceptions of the relative risk for transmission of HIV are different for each of the behaviors in question. A scale for each behavior in question should be constructed. Increase in the specificity of the measure increases the precision of the measurement (statistical power is discussed in greater detail in Chapter 9, and scaling, in Chapter 6).

Assessment of long-term behavioral changes is crucial to determining whether a program's overall goals are being met. As such, behavioral assessments immediately following multisessioned interventions are, at best, speculative regarding the extent to which participants maintain immediate benefits of participation over time. Monitoring participants over longer periods of time is essential to determine long-term behavior change.

Outcome Evaluation

Outcome evaluation refers to program effectiveness as it relates to the overall goal or purpose of an intervention. For example, educational efforts aimed at eliminating smoking are intended to reduce the incidence of lung cancer and heart disease. Impact evaluation would address whether the measurable objectives of the program have been met. For example, did 100% of the participants increase their knowledge about the health risks associated with smoking? Did 85% of the participants quit smoking for 3 months as a result of participation in the program? As noted earlier, impact evaluation is concerned with determining the effectiveness of a program on the actual program participants. Follow-up assessments are usually in close proximity (up to 2 years) to the intervention.

Outcome evaluation in health-related prevention programs tends to be long-term and medically based. The outcome of a smoking cessation initiative addresses the degree to which the goals of the program have been met. Did the rates of lung cancer and heart disease decrease for the community? The long-term nature of outcome evaluation makes it a costly form of evaluation.

Measures of morbidity and mortality are typically used as indicators of success in the outcome evaluation. As an overall goal, prevention programs focused on HIV-associated risk behaviors are designed to reduce the incidence of HIV infection in the targeted groups. Reduction in rates of seroconversion among participants (as compared to similar groups who have not received the intervention) has served as the primary index of program success. This would appear to be a reasonable indicator of outcome success, given that a goal of prevention is to stop the transmission of HIV. However, the cause of the reduction of incidence is not always clearcut. For example, in Uganda, the rate of HIV infection has decreased among teenagers over the past 5 years, and pregnant women testing positive has dropped from nearly 30% in some urban areas to 15–20% in the same time period (McKinley, 1996). It remains unknown whether this downward trend is because of actual large-scale behavioral change in the population due to intense prevention efforts or is an artifact due to the high death rate in this population.

Reduction in rates of STDs has also been used as an outcome measure of behavioral change. Demand for condoms, as measured by sales, is another indicator of HIV risk-reduction behavior. In pediatric–maternal HIV prevention programs, the overall goal is the reduction of the incidence of perinatal HIV transmission.

Because of the long incubation period between asymptomatic infection and the onset of clinical disease (9–10 years), using AIDS incidence rates as criteria for program success requires long-term monitoring within a community. Further, adequate data of population-based HIV infection rates cannot be obtained in many communities. In communities that have low HIV infection rates, too much time might elapse before sufficient numbers of cases are accrued; therefore, HIV seroincidence would not be a useful indicator of program effectiveness (Coyle *et al.*, 1991).

Using HIV seroconversion (change from being HIV-negative to HIV-positive) rates as outcome criteria in communities that have already experienced substantial behavioral change, such as self-identified gay and bisexual men in New York and San Francisco, may be misleading because of the difficulty in detecting intervention effects. For example, if participants increased condom use during receptive anal intercourse and their number of sexual partners per year prior to beginning the program, these extensive changes could diminish what might have occurred as a result of the intervention. At best, we can do no more than estimate such changes. Knowledge of a community or population's seroprevalence rate, however, can prioritize the need for risk-reducing interventions.

AIDS case rates do not reflect the current pattern of infection in a community, and given the period between infection and the development of AIDS, they are not appropriate indicators of behavioral change. Consequently, we often have to rely on more intermediate indicators of program success, such as improvements in knowledge, increased condom use, and maintenance of behavioral change.

Due to the complexity and expense associated with outcome evaluation, there have been few done in relation to HIV/AIDS prevention interventions. One noteworthy attempt has been the America Responds to AIDS campaign. This is a national media campaign designed to raise awareness about HIV/AIDS and to reduce its incidence in the general population through public service announcements (PSA) and print media. Outcome evaluation utilized changing trends in the awareness of HIV/AIDS, using a sample from the National Health Interview Survey. Seven new items were added to assess the impact of the national mailing of the brochure, *Understanding AIDS*, which comprised phase II of the campaign. Results of the survey indicated that 63% of the sample had received the brochure, at least half of those who received it read it, and it was discussed in one third of the households where the information was read (Coyle *et al.*, 1991). Monitoring national AIDS hotline calls is another means of determining increased awareness related to the pattern of PSA airings. In future phases of the campaign, PSAs will be aired aimed at specific segments of the population, e.g., adolescents. Increases in calls from adolescents to the National AIDS Hotline are one means of monitoring the longer-term effectiveness of the intervention.

In any event, this is not an inexpensive undertaking. It has been estimated that to conduct a national survey with a sample of 5000 respondents at three points in time could cost anywhere from $500,000 to $750,000. It is apparent that few organizations would be capable of executing such an outcome evaluation. In addition, it is unrealistic to presume that the implementation of a single intervention would result in significant changes in outcome variables such as seroprevalence, condom sales, or incidence of STDs. The role of the AIDS service organization and CBO in outcome evaluation is in the examination of the incremental contribution of a series of interventions implemented in the commu-

---

Example 3.3. Evaluation Issues for Project Reach

Project REACH is a public health education program in which residents of shelters for the homeless provide HIV/AIDS risk-reduction education to their fellow residents. This program was conceived and implemented with the assistance of a program evaluator. Process, impact, and outcome evaluation issues in determining the needs of the program and program content and in bringing the program to the residents were addressed prior to implementation. The major evaluation issues confronted by Project REACH, over time, are described below.

Issues	Process evaluation	Impact evaluation	Outcome evaluation
Research questions posed	• What are the needs of the shelter residents? • How will the program fit in with the operation of the shelter? • Was the projected number of residents served?	• Has the program increased the use of condoms among the residents? • Has the residents' level of AIDS-related knowledge increased?	• Is there a reduction in HIV seroconversion among the homeless? • Has the level of AIDS awareness risen among the homeless?
Indicators/ measures employed	• Needs assessment surveys • Interviews with residents • Focus groups with staff	• Self-administered knowledge questionnaires • Interviews with participants • Diaries	• Stabilized HIV seroconversion rate • Reduction in "dirty" urines among the homeless
Types of results	Qualitative— primarily	Quantitative— primarily	Quantitative— primarily
Utility of findings	• Determines program content • Modifies program content and implementation • Provides documentation for replicability of program	• Summative; indicates the degree to which program objectives have been met • Provides input to future implementation of program	• Determines overall effectiveness of program • Provides community with feedback on value of education
Who does it?	• Evaluation staff • Shelter staff • Shelter residents	• Health educators • Program participants	• Evaluators and interviewers • Total shelter population

(SOURCE: DiVittis & Badillo, 1994.)

nity. These interventions become part of an intervention strategy, targeted to specific segments of the population and timed for maximal effect. Through proper documentation of the implementation of the programs and impact evaluation of the intervention on the participants, organizations will have the raw data necessary to assess the outcome of an intervention strategy. The development of a peer education program in New York City's homeless shelters gives a composite view of some of the issues associated with the process, impact, and outcome evaluation of a prevention intervention (see Example 3.3).

Dissemination of Results

Many audiences express interest in the results of process and summative evaluations. The community in question needs such information to reinforce the work they have already done and to plan for the future needs of their constituents. Dissemination of these results often enable health care providers and public health officials to commit valuable resources in needed areas. Data from outcome evaluation are used by researchers, planners, funding sources, and government agencies to demonstrate a program's cost-effectiveness. It is important to keep in mind that the audience is broad based and that study findings must be tailored to the recipients' needs.

In order for evaluation results to be of value to a community, the organization, funder, and public health community, their dissemination must be timely. Further, information must be accessible. Alternative venues for publication of printed articles in professional journals are needed. Presentations at local community boards and at grand rounds in area hospitals are means of getting the word out to community leaders and health care providers. By publishing one's own newsletter, the evaluator maintains ongoing communication with his or her constituency and can provide them with timely updates. Finally, with the opening of the information superhighway, computer-based venues are another source of information dissemination. The use of computer bulletin boards and information clearinghouses can allow for instant access to evaluation results.

CONCLUSION

In general, program evaluation consists of techniques and tools that enable a person to determine the fit of the program to community needs, the implementation of the program, means of improving the program, and the short- and long-term results of the program. These tools seek to answer evaluation questions that will satisfy the needs of programmers and funders and offer something back to the community. The quality of the evaluation is also judged by how well the evaluators have sampled relevant content areas to be measured (e.g., knowledge, attitudes, and behaviors). The need to assess the process issues (formative and implementation) of the intervention as well as the effectiveness of the intervention (impact and outcome) will be illustrated in Chapter 9. These illustrations will show how AIDS service organizations with limited resources will be able to incorporate some evaluation strategies into their intervention programs.

As will be seen in subsequent chapters, the unique pressures of an HIV preventive intervention require the application and development of evaluation strategies that are scientifically objective and also responsive to the needs of the community.

Table 4.1. Issues for Consideration in a Needs Assessment

Dimension	Issues
Historical context	Have other needs assessments been conducted? Were they HIV/AIDS specific? What were the results of the needs assessment? What have been the barriers to collecting this type of information? What was the cost? Is it possible to use experienced personnel and community resources as consultants or workers?
Time line	When must the needs assessment be completed for useful decision making in program development and implementation?
Identification of community leaders and development of linkages	Who are the religious leaders, members of the school board, politicians, etc? What techniques are best for identifying community leaders (both individuals and members of organizations?) Have cohesive networks been developed for other projects, either AIDS- or non-AIDS-related? How can vested interest groups and community decision makers share information, build coalitions, develop task forces, and be involved in the needs assessment? How can these coalitions work together in the future?
Role assignments	Who will be responsible within the community for the various tasks in the needs assessment? What role will each organization play with other community organizations?
Planning of data collection	Can existing qualitative and quantitative data be used? What additional data should be collected? Which data collection methods are most appropriate with respect to usability, time, cost-benefits, trained personnel, and community acceptability?
Preplanning	Has appropriate time been built into the needs-assessment plan? What are the anticipated barriers to conducting a needs assessment? How can they be overcome? Is there a contingency plan?
Resource constraints	What are the limitations of data collection due to constraints on community participation, time, money, and personnel?
Priorities of needs	By what criteria will community needs be prioritized? How does the availability of financial resources affect prioritization of needs? What will be the relative weight of felt vs. real needs, qualitative vs. quantitative data, subgroup vs. larger community, prevention vs. chronic illness, impact vs. outcome?
Ethical considerations	What are the ethical issues involved in a needs assessment? How will they be conveyed to the community? How will confidentiality and privacy be assured? What mechanisms can be put in place to address the potential for a community's elevated level of expectations and the possibility of negative outcomes? What concerns do community members have about the ethics of the evaluation team, choice of research methods, and the ways in which the data will be interpreted?
Dissemination of information	How will results of the needs assessment be disseminated to individuals and organizations within the community as well as to government officials and funders?

The HIV/AIDS intervention and evaluation team needs to know not only who currently lives in the community, but its social, economic, and medical history. What are the current HIV/AIDS policies and programs and how did they develop? Are community residents aware of the HIV/AIDS-related education programs and services in their community? If not, what types of educational interventions can facilitate this awareness? Table 4.2 identifies areas to be considered for gathering HIV/AIDS information and the questions that should be posed in collecting needs assessment or community analysis data.

Table 4.2. Domains for Community Assessment for Development and Evaluation of HIV/AIDS Preventive Interventions

Domain	Description of indicators
Sociodemographics	Age, gender, race, ethnic identity and acculturation, sexual orientation, socioeconomic status, immigration status
Social, economic, and political history	Organizational and political structural relationships that exist among community members as well as between social institutions and policymakers at the local, city, state, and federal level
	Social, economic, and political trends, e.g., unemployment, crime, and victimization
Comparison of major causes of disease and HIV/AIDS	Statistics on major causes and rates of morbidity, disability, infant and adult mortality
	Statistics on spectrum of HIV infection and AIDS-related mortality
	Comparison of statistics from target community with those of larger metropolitan region, state, and nation
Health care services and HIV/AIDS services	Health care services that exist in the community and those used outside of the community
	Perceived barriers to quality health care; competition among services for existing resources
	Community relationships with health care institutions and practitioners
	Availability of HIV-specific services (e.g., HIV counseling and testing and supportive follow-up services, mental health, drug treatment, TB, STDs, and maternal health care programs)
HIV/AIDS risk factors and impact	Risk factors for HIV infection
	Incidence and prevalence of HIV/AIDS delineated by age, gender, race, ethnicity, sexual orientation, and secular trends
	Impact on social, economic, and political life of the community
HIV/AIDS knowledge and attitudes	Level of HIV/AIDS knowledge in community
	Sources of information (e.g., family, friends, health providers, traditional healers, media)
	Community standards and norms
	Community and individual beliefs about causes and prevention of HIV and attitudes toward persons with HIV/AIDS
Prioritization of HIV/AIDS services	Prioritizing of HIV-related vs. non-HIV-related health and social service programs (e.g., media awareness campaigns, prevention education programs targeted to sexual behavior or drug use, therapies)
	Services available for community members, number of health care providers, and health and social organizations providing HIV-related services
	Programs and services to be altered, improved, or eliminated
HIV/AIDS policies	Existence of HIV/AIDS policies established by local and state entities, such as the health department, public assistance program, school board, home health care agencies, Medicaid/Medi-Cal, and national organizations, such as Social Security and third-party insurers. These policies might address hospital stay and use of other health care facilities, insurance benefits, medical personnel, HIV testing and serostatus, and HIV-infected patients with TB
	Rationale for existence or non-existence of particular policies

To assure a complete and successful community needs assessment, many types of information must be collected from the target population. Within the targeted group, gatekeepers of the information must be identified and their participation solicited. Gatekeepers include the "professionals" (e.g., health educators, health counselors, clinical and social service providers), "formal community leaders" (e.g., members of community boards, local politicians), and the "informal community leaders" (e.g., active church members, drug pushers, etc.) within the community.

Once the groups have been identified, information is gathered, using a variety of methods. The methods listed in Table 4.3 represent the most commonly used techniques and types of information to be gathered.

A community analysis can be conducted, using all or some of the aforementioned techniques. Often, program planners and evaluators are limited by funding, lead time, or trained personnel and volunteers. Because time and resources are often scarce, it may be cost-effective to use existing statistical data rather than collect new data.

The unit of analysis in a community needs assessment can vary—from the entire population in a geographic area to a segment of the population based on specific demographics or employees within a particular organization. To encourage persons and agencies to participate, there must be a match between the types of assessment tools and the environments in which assessment takes place. Example 4.1 briefly describes two needs assessments targeted toward women conducted at a conference and a health club, which incorporate varied data collection methods.

One popular application of needs assessment is to determine baseline knowledge, attitudes, and behaviors about sex, drug use, contraception, and preventive health practices. For example, the National Center for Health Statistics' quantitative survey data of knowledge and attitudes about HIV/AIDS among various subgroups of the US population can serve as the basis for planning for targeted nationwide campaigns to increase knowledge of HIV-related risk behaviors.

Needs assessment research is not limited to quantitative methods. Qualitative methods can provide information about the magnitude of a problem. For example, surveys of injection drug users, along with small-group interviews with primary sex partners of injection drug users, may yield important information about barriers to condom use. Qualitative strategies, such as ethnographic interviews, key informant interviews, and participant observation, are discussed in Chapter 7.

The four case studies that follow illustrate the use of needs assessment as part of the formative evaluation process. They address the varied populations that can benefit from a community analysis, the diverse settings for obtaining information, and the multimethod approach used to identify community needs. By using a multimethod approach, the needs assessment of gay and bisexual men investigates the current services and interventions for this population on a national basis. Two studies address the needs of gay and bisexual men of color—one conducted in a bar and the other by the US Conference of Mayors. The Association for Women's AIDS Research and Education's (AWARE) needs assessment highlights women's concerns about HIV and a timely feedback loop. Through the experience of conducting this analysis, AWARE was able to facilitate a similar study for COYOTE (a sex workers' rights organization). Often, staff at community-based organizations assess the needs of the target populations in the external community, but neglect

Table 4.3. Advantages and Disadvantages of Different
Needs Assessment Data Collection Techniques

Source of information	Advantages	Limitations
Secondary data sources (US Census, Centers for Disease Control and Prevention, National Center for Health Statistics, local and state health departments, hospitals, family planning, and other health and service agencies)	Provides sociodemographic information on AIDS cases, contraceptive use, unintended pregnancies, drug use, physical location, housing, employment, income, household characteristics, and education levels Reports incidence and prevalence data as well as statistics on birth, disability, morbidity, and infant and adult mortality	Geographic boundaries for data collection areas such as census tract, zip code, and community districts are often inconsistent Data are not always collected in consistent intervals Census data undercount the homeless and undocumented immigrants; data are often out of date due to its collection interval of every 10 years Data are not released on timely basis Data across organizations are inconsistent given variety of methods of collection and reporting
Literature review (e.g., *Health Education Quarterly, Health Education Research, American Journal of Public Health, Journal of Adolescent Health, Journal of Sex Research, AIDS Education and Prevention, AIDS, New England Journal of Medicine*, and other published sources)	Provides the names of program planners and evaluators Identifies empirically tested research instruments and techniques Describes successful and ineffective programs Recommends future research questions and areas for further inquiry Relatively low cost	Provides information bound to the samples tested and may not necessarily relate to the community for which your intervention is intended Published on the basis of statistical significance, which may not relate to "real world" desired changes in behavior Time lags in submission and publication can result in out-of-date information
Record utilization review/archival research (e.g., patient charts, hospital records, clinic records, HIV counseling and testing site records, certificates, toxicology reports)	Existing data base Data from charts or records document numbers of persons with a specific condition and those who have received education, services, treatment and counseling Provides data on secular trends Data are maintained according to a set of institutional standards	No community input Reluctance of health care providers and organizations to share information Confidentiality and anonymity can be compromised Inconsistency within and among organizations in quality of data recording Data may be hard to read or incomplete Time-consuming, labor-intensive process Costs vary by expertise of reviewer (e.g., nurse vs. student)
Community survey	Allows for direct input from community Can be used as marketing technique to increase community awareness of project	High cost of trained interviewers Cost of incentives for participants Survey sample may not be representative of community

(continued)

Table 4.3. (*Continued*)

Source of Information	Advantages	Limitations
Face-to-face interview	Can stratify by population (e.g., service providers, men of color, gay/bisexual men, IDUs) Provides timely identification of needs Can clarify questions through interviewer–participant interaction	Can be relatively expensive if expert services are not donated or if community conducts its own survey
Telephone survey	Easy to administer Low cost Large outreach	Bias in response rate—significant proportions of the target population may not have phones or may refuse to participate in the survey; conversation may be constrained by lack of privacy
Mailed questionnaire	Easy to administer Relatively low cost Large outreach	Low response rate results in bias Access to mailing lists
Opinion leader's survey (e.g., religious, political, social service)	Knowledgeable source is reporting on community Smaller sample than population-based survey	May not represent all community points of view Subjective point of view
Key informant Members of the community who are identified as "knowledgeable" due to respect, history in the community (e.g., *bodega* owners, beauticians, long-time residents)	Little cost, time, and resources required Focuses needs assessment on precise issues Facilitates networking among human services, health agencies, and politicians Develops a group to collaborate during program planning, implementation, and evaluation	Should be used only in conjunction with other methods; if not, information may be skewed Subjective viewpoint Potentially incorporates professional biases Does not represent all subgroups within the community
Community forum	Relatively easy to arrange Inexpensive compared to other needs assessment methods Useful for identifying individuals interested in the specific topic area	Impossible to assure representation of all views Least empowered often will not be represented Participants may not want to reveal their feelings due to fear of retaliation Can deteriorate into complaint session Participants' expectations may be raised without the ability to meet expectations
Focus groups	Identifies concerns of community members Considered an essential method for gaining information from HIV-infected persons Relatively easy to develop instruments Inexpensive Results can be available within a short time	Results are hard to quantify Trained personnel needed to facilitate groups Participants may be typical but not representative of community members Generalizability of results contingent on how well the sample represents the community

---

Example 4.1. Using Small-Group Process and Surveys
to Determine a Community's Needs

The National Hemophilia Foundation

While the National Hemophilia Foundation (NHF) had concentrated on AIDS
prevention, diagnosis, and care needs of male hemophiliacs, women as partners,
mothers, patients (von Willebrand disease or bleeding disorder) and caregivers are also
affected by the illness. Employees at the national office and women throughout the
country worked to develop a needs-assessment/education program. In October 1989,
women from each region of the country were flown free of charge to a weekend
conference. The conference was developed by a panel of NHF employees, hemophilia
community members, and professionals, including anthropologists, physicians, psychol-
ogists, and health educators. Assessment of needs was made through the use of focus
groups, role plays, and written recommendations. A list of women and their phone
numbers was provided to foster social support networks following the conference. A
newsletter was developed, and plans for action around health insurance, support of
school personnel, and development of an ongoing organization were made. Through
needs assessment, the needed role models, health care professionals, social support
networks, communication outlets, and action strategies to mobilize and maintain a
women's organization were put into place. (From Auerbach, 1995, Hunter College,
School of Health Sciences, personal communication.)

The San Francisco AIDS Foundation

The San Francisco AIDS Foundation conducted a series of surveys that showed that
heterosexual women in San Francisco, while denying their personal risk, engaged in
behaviors that put them at risk for HIV. Prior to implementing community-based AIDS
prevention workshops for women, a needs assessment instrument was distributed at
health clubs to determine what women knew about AIDS and their attitudes about
workshops. The survey sampled such domains as:

- Knowledge about transmission (e.g., How do women get AIDS?)
- Prevention techniques (e.g., What is safe sex?)
- Negotiation (e.g., How can women start to talk about safe sex with their
  partners?)
- Communication (e.g., How can women talk about AIDS with their teenage or
  adult children?)
- Self-perceived risk (e.g., Are you worried about you? your sex partner? your
  children?)
- Desire to participate in a workshop (e.g., Would you attend a free workshop to
  get answers to your questions?)

(SOURCE: Auerbach, 1988.)

to assess the needs of the volunteers. The Gay Men's Health Crisis case study addresses satisfaction and stresses, as well as ways to educate and support volunteers to be more successful in their work with clients and the public.

CASE STUDY OF US CONFERENCE OF MAYORS: GAY AND BISEXUAL MEN OF COLOR

The Problem

Despite greater funding for targeted HIV prevention and service delivery networks, these initiatives were not meeting the needs of the gay male communities of color. Even with stabilizing rates of HIV infection in the gay community as a whole, rates continued to escalate among gay and bisexual men of color, who accounted for the more than 20% of the total cumulative AIDS cases in the United States. This was documented by reported statistics from 2 years' earlier that showed men of color accounted for 35% of all newly identified cases of AIDS in gay and bisexual men.

Evaluation Strategy

To understand why the numbers of HIV-infected minority gay men were increasing, a comprehensive needs assessment was conducted of African-American, Hispanic, Asian and Pacific Islander, and Native-American gay and bisexual communities in five cities (Chicago, Los Angeles, New York City, Oklahoma City, and San Juan, Puerto Rico). Multiple sources of data collection, which combined qualitative and quantitative methods, were used to ascertain the viewpoint of service providers and describe members of the gay and bisexual communities.

Data Collection Methods

Literature Review. Consultants reviewed the instruments and results of published studies that assessed the knowledge, attitudes, beliefs, and behavior of gay and bisexual men of color. This information was used to develop appropriate evaluation strategies and tools.

Primary Prevention Service Provider Surveys. Organizations that provided HIV prevention services were surveyed to assess types of programs, budgets, number and type of staff, volunteers representative of the target population, staff's language abilities, and quality of community linkages with gay and bisexual men of color.

Key Community Informant Interviews. Community leaders of gay or AIDS agencies, policymakers, and advocates were given semistructured interviews that addressed HIV prevention needs of gay and bisexual men of color, the cultural appropriateness of community responses to those needs, and experiences with local health departments.

Target Population Recruitment. Outreach workers identified men who could benefit from primary prevention services, particularly those who did not know their HIV status or who were HIV-negative. Snowball sampling, in which research participants recommend other potential participants to contact for study participation, was used to identify members of friendship networks and participants in gay events to advertise the study. Sample recruitment was based on characteristics such as age, race, ethnicity, socioeconomic level, education, and language spoken.

Open-Ended Interviews. Trained interviewers taped conversations with participants. Areas of discussion included the impact of HIV, personal experiences with health and social services, and social and family support.

Structured Questionnaires. Questionnaires administered by trained interviewers addressed sexual orientation, knowledge, attitudes, beliefs and behaviors about HIV, safer sex and drugs, access to HIV prevention services and care, and the impact of HIV on social support networks.

Focus Groups. Outreach was conducted by a project coordinator and representatives from CBOs to facilitate representation from the four ethnic groups. The nominal group process (which provides equal voting power to each participant) was used to conduct ethnic-specific focus groups. Each group was asked: "What needs to be done in (city) among (ethnic) men whose sexual behavior is like yours to decrease the spread of HIV?"

Local Health Department and State AIDS Information. Using a standardized questionnaire, local health department and state representatives were asked for assistance in compiling HIV seroprevalence, funding levels for HIV prevention programs, the kinds and numbers of programs they presented or contracted out, and technical assistance needs. Those interviewed ranged from epidemiologists to grants managers.

Results

Interview and questionnaire data from 285 gay and bisexual men of color, 42 key informants, 300 primary prevention service providers, 7 staff members from each local health department, and 5 state AIDS coordinators, highlighted the need for more HIV prevention services directed to gay and bisexual men of color, especially Native Americans, Asian and Pacific Islanders, and adolescents. Only New York City had specific programs for gay and bisexual men of color. While New York and Los Angeles had fairly well-established services and organizations, there was a special need in communities that lacked gay minority organizations, outreach activities, networks, and social support groups. Services for Native Americans and Asian and Pacific Islanders were meager, possibly due to their diversity of cultures and languages. The lack of health care providers who spoke their native languages and printed materials in native languages contributed to the gap in HIV/AIDS prevention programs and services.

The study also highlighted a severe lack of targeted HIV/AIDS prevention programs, gay minority organizations, networks, support groups, and outreach activities for this population. Fortunately, the efforts of the study participants and results of the community needs assessment of the five cities were recognized for their contribution to this area of study. Based on the identified need, the US Conference of Mayors issued a request for proposals to implement HIV preventive interventions for gay men of color. Twenty applications were received and $70,000 was given to three organizations to fund responsive programs that would develop networking and sharing of resources between local health departments and community-based agencies (US Conference of Mayors, 1994).

This case study illustrates the process by which needs in diverse communities across many settings can be identified and appropriate actions taken to meet those needs. By approaching the problem from a variety of sources and using a variety of methods, an evaluator is able to build in validation of the community assessment by finding agreement across the methods/sources of data (referred to as triangulation). To maximize results for the communities in need, a health educator and evaluator will need to tap these sources of information continually throughout the program planning, implementation, and evaluation processes.

A thorough plan for community needs assessment can enhance the development of a program that is sensitive, timely, and appropriate for the target population. The case study of AWARE illustrates the importance of community coalition building in the assessment of a community's needs, development of research questions and protocols, and intervention implementation (Cohen, Derish, & Dorfman, 1994).

CASE STUDY OF THE ASSOCIATION FOR WOMEN'S AIDS RESEARCH AND EDUCATION

The Problem

In 1984, AWARE was founded to perform an epidemiological study of the prevalence of HIV infection among women in San Francisco. This was at a time when little was known about HIV infection among women outside of injection drug use and transfusion-related transmission. Heterosexual transmission was not a recognized risk factor. Given the diversity of women at risk (e.g., sex workers, injection drug use, monogamous women, women with multiple sex partners), that many women were unaware of their HIV risk, and the sensitive nature of the questions (illicit drug use and sexual behaviors), identifying the "community" to be surveyed became a formidable task. It was safe to say that this represented a "hard-to-reach" population.

Evaluation Strategy

The first step that the AWARE researchers undertook was to identify the community to be studied. This was accomplished by holding open meetings in which women from the community could participate. Through these discussions, the researchers were able to address the concerns of the women of San Francisco and incorporate those concerns into a research design.

Some of the issues addressed were:

- Women did not want to feel like guinea pigs, providing information and receiving nothing in return. To ensure that this was not the case, researchers made services available to participants and released results of the study in a timely manner to the community and through presentations at professional conferences.
- Interview instruments were constructed with wording in the participants' own language.
- Multiple interview sites were identified around the city where women from a variety of risk backgrounds could feel comfortable. These sites included public and private clinics, drug treatment facilities, residence hotels, and a large county hospital.
- Interviewers were hired from these sites to provide a point of identification for the participant. By having regular staff conduct the interviews, participant confidentiality was protected. In this way, women could come for "regular" services and not necessarily be identified as participants in an HIV/AIDS study.

Results

By including the input of the community and providing feedback, AWARE was able to identify and engage a community of women at risk for HIV infection, obtain necessary epidemiological data, and provide educational and health services to the women in need. The success of this model was repeated in 1985 when AWARE joined COYOTE (a sex workers' rights organization) to conduct a similar epidemiological study among San Francisco sex workers. Through an open dialogue between the researchers and the sex workers, a culturally competent research protocol was developed. The interviewers were former sex workers who were trained to engage women on the streets, recruit them for participation, interview them, and even draw their blood for testing.

Results of the study demonstrated that sex workers were not the "vectors of disease" that many politicians had assumed. In fact, HIV/AIDS had strengthened the long-time practice of condom use with customers. As with the first study, the linkages between community members and the professional health evaluation team provided a realistic approach to the needs of the community and the research itself. This is the initial step in developing goals and objectives, program activities, and implementation of an HIV/AIDS intervention (Cohen *et al.*, 1994).

CASE STUDY OF GAY MEN'S HEALTH CRISIS SUPPORT NETWORK PROJECT

The Problem

It is often difficult to assess the educational needs of isolated populations. In 1993, Gay Men's Health Crisis developed the Informational and Support Network Project to analyze how HIV/AIDS information is transmitted through personal networks of African-American and Latino men who have sex with men in Queens (Jackson Heights and Elmhurst), New York. To gain background information to design a community-level peer mobilization intervention, a needs assessment was conducted.

Evaluation Strategy

Structured anonymous interviews were conducted with 157 men from the targeted communities. These interviews were conducted in bars and community-based organizations within the target area. Questions addressed demographics, transculturation (the process whereby an individual is actively adapting to and influencing the dominant culture), knowledge about HIV/AIDS, intentions and barriers to practicing safer sex, and frequency of protected anal and oral sex.

Results

Differences were found between men who were born in the United States and those born in Latin America. Among all men who had engaged in anal intercourse in the previous 2 months, only 52% reported always using a condom. Factors associated with protected insertive anal sex were intentions to practice safer sex and negative expectations about acting safely. Engaging in protective anal sex was more likely for men born in South America. Respondents who intended to engage in protected insertive anal sex were more likely to practice safer sex. Protected oral sex was associated with HIV/AIDS knowledge and intention to practice safer sex. Differences in individual-level variables associated with distinct behaviors should be targeted in community-based interventions programs. The unique cultural aspects of the many nationalities that constitute the Latino community should be considered when developing community needs assessment recruitment techniques as well as developing HIV/AIDS education. In addition, socioeconomic status needs to be considered, since it is a powerful predictor of protected anal and protected oral sex (Cairo, Genaro, Whittier, & Miller, 1994, 1995).

CASE STUDY OF GAY MEN'S HEALTH CRISIS EDUCATION DEPARTMENT VOLUNTEERS

Often, health care organizations evaluate the needs of employees at ongoing meetings with supervisors or annual reviews. The majority of AIDS-related community-based agencies, particularly those that provide counseling and education, have large volunteer staffs that do not have structured forums for feedback. Education program volunteers represent the agency while working directly with persons needing primary prevention and those who are receiving health care services. To provide and maintain a high level of positive educational experiences, it is essential to have a satisfied and empowered volunteer staff. The following case study describes a needs assessment of volunteers in the education department of GMHC.

Evaluation Strategy

During Fall 1991 and Winter 1992, GMHC conducted a needs assessment of its education department volunteers to determine whether volunteer needs had been met, how to optimize volunteer satisfaction, and therefore increase volunteer retention and program quality. The volunteer study addressed volunteers' motivation, satisfaction, and stress. Earlier studies of paid workers found job stress had a negative effect on satisfaction (Holt, 1982; Porter & Steers, 1973; Schuh, 1967). GMHC wanted to assess the prevalence of volunteer stress in all volunteer job categories. By identifying stressors, supervisors could possibly restructure jobs to be less stressful.

Data Collection Method

A pool of 294 eligible participants was identified from the list of education department volunteers (i.e., those who had volunteered during the past year). Volunteers were mailed a letter announcing a survey. One week later, they received a follow-up phone call from a Hunter College Master of Public Health student intern to encourage participation in the survey. Anonymity in survey responses was guaranteed.

One week following the phone call, each volunteer received a questionnaire, a self-addressed, stamped envelope, and, as an incentive, a raffle entry card for a pair of free tickets to a circus event sponsored by GMHC. This questionnaire, which incorporated both open-ended and closed-ended items, was constructed after pretesting on a similar population. Reminders to return the questionnaires were sent 2 and 4 weeks following the initial mailing. Of the 294 questionnaires mailed, 27 were returned as undeliverable. Among those, correct addresses were found for 18 volunteers. A total of 172 responses (a 60% response rate) were received.

Limitations

Due to the anonymity of the questionnaires, there was no way to identify characteristics of the volunteers who responded from those who did not respond. It was also impossible to ascertain if the respondents were representative of the larger education department volunteer pool. By surveying only currently active volunteers, the reasons for volunteers' inactivity or dropout from the program were unknown.

Results

Satisfaction

Respondents worked in 14 program areas. About 63% of the volunteers reported that their expectations were "very much" met, while about 28% had "some degree" of met expectations. Job type was significantly related to satisfaction. Speakers (those who provided public speaking and group facilitation) were more satisfied than administrative assistants (those who worked with data and materials or provided administrative support); counselors (those who provided information, support, and referrals in one-on-one interaction) were more satisfied than both administrative assistants and outreach workers (those who went to communities to provide basic information and materials). The average satisfaction score ranged from "very satisfied" to "some." Counselors were the most satisfied of groups, while administrative assistants were the least satisfied. Volunteer satisfaction was unrelated to stress, either in number of stressors or how burdensome they were.

Stress

More than 75% of volunteers experienced stress when having to think about poor people, having heard unpleasant remarks about GMHC, and learning a volunteer co-worker was HIV-positive. When asked to respond to an open-ended question about a stressful event they had encountered in volunteering, they described interactions with clients who had many problems, such as poor health, poverty, homelessness, unemployment, and no access to health care. There was no difference in the overall number of stressors experienced by job type, but these stressors varied by job type. Speakers were most likely to encounter racism, homophobia, and comments about persons with AIDS "deserving it." They were also the most likely to experience being nervous in their job. Counselors felt most empowered about their ability to complete tasks.

Workplace Climate

Volunteers rated the workplace climate high, particularly on the supportiveness of staff and other volunteers, involvement in department life, and procedures for volunteers. Volunteers who perceived a high level of job orientation were most satisfied as were those who felt a departmental cohesion. Routine jobs were seen as less rewarding, while spontaneous interaction with the public was seen as more rewarding.

The results of this needs assessment indicated that supervisors should place more emphasis on organization through well-defined tasks and encourage volunteers to be creative and spontaneous in the completion of these tasks. Wherever possible, cohesion with other volunteers should be facilitated through the use of the team approach. Working with clients in a one-to-one situation should be encouraged for all volunteers, which may include expanding the variety of roles individual volunteers play. Expanded training to address issues of poverty and its related social, economic, and medical problems is necessary to alleviate some of the stress encountered by education volunteers (Miller, Holmes, & Auerbach, 1992).

SHARING RESULTS OF THE NEEDS ASSESSMENT

An essential part of the evaluation process is sharing the results of the needs assessment not only with funders but also with the community that has been analyzed. Community-based agencies, health care organizations, schools, and volunteers who have participated in the process will anticipate receiving the findings. A written report, no matter how simple, can enhance the discussion between the community and those responsible for the interventions. Planners and evaluators should communicate findings in a manner that reflects the mission of the organization, the size and severity of the problems, and the gaps between problems and appropriate services to ameliorate them. Distributing a report prior to a community forum affords recipients the time to review the results, form questions, and develop specific recommendations. A community forum will allow participants to obtain immediate feedback from the evaluation team and to hear from and share comments with others. Observers' notes and audio or videotaping of the forum will provide documentation of participant feedback that can be used to inform future interventions. Another inexpensive feedback mechanism is the use of suggestion boxes at health and social institutions or stores.

NEEDS ASSESSMENT AS AN ONGOING PROCESS

After the needs assessment, dissemination of findings, and interventions have been put in place, the community analysis process is not complete. Because a community is not a static entity, a community's needs should be assessed periodically. Various factors can impact a community, mandating an updated needs assessment. These factors include: (1) historical events that change a community; (2) changes in the science and policies of HIV/AIDS that necessitate new interventions; (3) implementation of the intervention that results in a changing of the community; and (4) community response to a need in the interim between the findings of the needs assessment and program developers' responses.

Following a needs assessment, the impact of an historical event can change the community. For example, the announcement that Magic Johnson is HIV-infected resulted in adolescents identifying with the possibility of infection. This, in turn, changed the awareness needs of adolescents targeted for HIV prevention intervention. In addition, as we learn more about the treatment and prevention of HIV infection, this creates new needs in the affected population. For example, the effectiveness of AIDS Clinical Trial Group (ACTG) protocol 076 in the prevention of maternal–infant HIV transmission with administration of zidovudine [formerly called azidothymidine (AZT)] to pregnant women has led to policy changes that range from the mandatory testing of pregnant women to the unblinding of newborn HIV screening results. With these changing policies, new needs have emerged among the affected population, including civil rights issues, balancing an effective medical intervention with reaching the women in greatest need of intervention (*New York Times*, 1996), and educational needs of the population most affected by these discoveries.

The implementation of successful interventions in a community may meet some needs and in turn create others. For example, an effective intervention that results in gay men negotiating for safer sex may meet an immediate prevention need in that population segment. Having met that need, an unmet need of relationship-building skills in the same population may be highlighted.

Delays between the needs assessment and funding of the program can result in the discovery that previously unmet needs have been met. For example, a needs assessment in New York City indicated that the homeless with tuberculosis and HIV infection were noncompliant with their directly observed therapy. To increase directly observed therapy

Table 5.1. Threats to Internal Validity

Type of threat	Description	Solution
History	Unanticipated events occurring between assessments, secular trends, e.g., changes in drug treatment philosophy, development of new policies regarding condom distribution within shelters.	1. Include items that assess respondent's experiences since last assessed (e.g., significant AIDS-related events). 2. Use a design that controls for history, such as cross-lag panel design. Here, new respondents serve as controls at each subsequent observation.
Maturation	Naturally occurring developmental changes within individuals, e.g., becoming older, more seasoned and experienced, being HIV infected.	1. Make testing periods relatively short. 2. Use interrupted time series design instead of pre- or posttest only designs.
Statistical regression	Samples with extreme behavior regress toward the overall group average, e.g., individuals with high levels of HIV-related knowledge may score lower at follow-up, while those with low baseline knowledge scores may score better at follow-up.	1. Statistically control by Windsorizing scores (eliminate extreme scores) or by using multiple measurement points and using an average. 2. Avoid recruiting participants with extreme low or high scores as study subjects. 3. Random assignment of participants to either experimental or control conditions.
Instrumentation	Changes in assessment tools, criteria or cutoffs for a specific behavior, e.g., for what is considered to be drug-positive or toxicity, over the course of evaluation.	It is important not to change instruments during the course of the study. In the event that this is impossible, e.g., having to change labs for drug testing, keep both the old and new labs for a period to determine equivalence before dropping the old lab.
Testing	Reactivity to repeated testing. Effects of repeated testing on subsequent testing (e.g., repeated test taking improves test-taking skills, which in turn improves scores).	Use multiple, equivalent forms of the same test, or use control (untested) groups to control statistically for reactivity.
Selection	Differences, e.g., social (availability of social support network), demographic, motivational, cognitive, attitudinal, between intervention and control group participants.	1. Determine the groups' equivalence at baseline and statistically control for differences in analysis. 2. Random assignment of participants to either experimental or control conditions. 3. Careful selection of participant inclusion criteria.
Sample attrition or experimental mortality	Differential dropout or mortality across the study period.	Analyze data on dropout participants to determine if there are any patterns that would limit generalizability of results.
Hawthorne effect	Effects found independent of intervention. Effect of being in a program or an evaluation.	Give comparison groups the intervention on a delayed testing basis to see if differential effects are found.

population (e.g., all residents in a homeless shelter) a number from the random numbers table. If your goal is to randomly select one tenth of the population of shelter residents, you could select everyone whose assigned number ended in five. On the average, this will result in the random selection of 10% of the population.

Stratified Random

Prior to selecting a sample, an evaluator subdivides the population into homogenous categories or strata. These characteristics are believed to be important to the representativeness of the sample. Stratifying the population minimizes differences within categories and maximizes these differences between. Participants are randomly selected from within each stratum. Sampling in this fashion then ensures that individuals with the characteristic of interest are represented in the sample. Demographic variables often serve as the basis for stratification. For example, in a study of the relationship between cultural factors and HIV sexual risk reduction among Latina immigrants, stratified sampling may be used to ensure that Dominicans, Mexicans, and Colombians are adequately represented in the sample. This is especially important if the evaluator believes that the proportion of Latina immigrants engaging in HIV risk behavior varies by national origin. This stratification may be in proportion to their representation in the population.

Sometimes, if a particular characteristic of a population occurs infrequently but is deemed important to the study, it will be sampled disproportionately or oversampled. For example, if African Americans are underrepresented in a population but disproportionately affected by HIV, you may want to include a larger proportion of them in the sample than represented in the population.

Systematic

With this method, participant names are selected from a list. The first name is chosen randomly, and then additional names are selected by taking every third, fourth, tenth, and so on name until the desired sample size is achieved. For example, if you want to select a systematic sample from a STD clinic, the list of patients waiting to be seen on particular days can easily be used. Other sources of lists that can be employed to draw a systematic sample include: college student roster, telephone books, organizational memberships, voter registration, and clinic patients in a hospital. The evaluator should be certain, however, that there is no inherent pattern in the sequence of names on the list. Also, the evaluator should be aware of biases associated with the source, e.g., all people do not have telephones; telephone lists are not representative of all those who have telephones; and not everyone is a registered voter.

Cluster

This method of sampling enables the evaluator to randomly identify participants when the total population is unknowable. With this method, the sampling unit is a group or cluster, such as churches, schools, classrooms, housing projects, factories, shelters, and census tracts, rather than individuals. The clusters are identified and randomly sampled, ensuring that a broad range of clusters are included. From the identified clusters, subgroups of clusters may be identified. When the smallest set of clusters are identified, a random sample of participants is drawn from the clusters. It is important to note that whenever any type of sample is drawn, there is always the chance for error. When more than one stage of sampling is applied (such as in cluster sampling), the probability of error increases with each additional stage.

Although it may be difficult to identify the population of women who deliver in hospitals in New York City, it is relatively easy to obtain a list of all hospitals in the city. From this first-stage cluster (all hospitals), the evaluator can stratify by hospital type (e.g., borough, public vs. private, size). From within each stratum (e.g., small public hospitals in Queens), a sample of hospitals is randomly selected (second-stage cluster). From within these hospitals, a random sample of women who delivered is drawn (third-stage cluster), representing a pool of participants eligible for inclusion in the evaluation. Depending on the needs of the evaluation, the sample can be further stratified from this identified pool of participants.

Nonprobability

In nonprobability samples, participants are selected for sample inclusion based on their accessibility. Not everyone in the population has an equal chance of being in the sample. Nonprobability samples can be drawn in several ways, as described.

Convenience

Samples of convenience are drawn on the basis of opportunity of participants. Participants are often members of an intact group. Examples of convenience samples include HIV-infected patients attending a clinic, subway riders, a class of college students, people in a shopping mall, gay and bisexual men on a beach, bar patrons, and women attending a women's festival. A major advantage of convenience samples is that a large amount of data can be collected relatively rapidly from a large number of people.

Although convenience samples are easy to recruit, this method provides the least amount of generalizability. For example, findings based on a sample of women who attend a women's festival are not representative of all women. However, because of practical considerations, evaluators often have to rely on this type of sampling. For example, samples of women who have sex with women are usually based on convenient access to self-identified lesbians because of the difficulty in discerning them in a population-based probability sample.

The rapid collection of information provides the evaluator with the ready means to generate hypotheses, identify issues of interest to the population, and obtain results that can be used in the implementation of more stringent experimental designs.

Snowball

Snowball sampling, also known as chain referral sampling, is especially useful when members of difficult-to-identify populations, such as male prostitutes, bisexual men, drag queens, and adolescents involved in high-risk activities, know one another. In a snowball sample, a small group of members of this population is initially identified by the researcher; these members then are asked to refer other members. Each new participant is then requested to name additional people. This iterative process continues until the desired sample size is achieved. The success of this type of sampling is dependent on the number of members' contacts with other members of that population. Socially isolated members of the population have a reduced chance of being included in the sample because they lack the initial contact for referral (Kalton, 1983). Like convenience sampling, the ability to make inferences to the general population is limited.

Quota

This approach is the nonprobability equivalent of the stratified random sample. With knowledge of the characteristics of the population, a matrix to identify the "strata" of interest is constructed. The evaluator then sets out to fill these quotas or strata. Here, the sample is drawn based on proportions of particular characteristics or variables, such as gender, race/ethnicity, and age. Unlike stratified random sampling, where the population is grouped into stratum and randomly sampled from within each group, in quota sampling the categories are created and filled later.

Sometimes, quotas of these characteristics reflect their population parameters. For example, with quota sampling on race/ethnicity, the proportion of African Americans and Latino/as may be based on the proportion of these groups in the local community or nationwide. Minority groups are often oversampled to give confidence that they represent their actual population parameters.

Errors associated with this sampling strategy include the problems of accurately constructing quotas that represent the population. Second, because a researcher does not have access to all members of the population within a quota, the sample obtained may not be representative of the group. For example, if your quota prescribes the inclusion of 12 Puerto Rican males, the ones selected to fill the quota may not be representative of males in the population of Puerto Ricans. To increase the likelihood of diversity, the quotas of interest can be oversampled.

RANDOMIZED EXPERIMENTAL VERSUS QUASI-EXPERIMENTAL DESIGNS

Randomized experimental designs are the gold standard of research. They imply that the researcher has complete control over all of the conditions of the experiment. The experimental design incorporates a group that receives the experimental treatment, an equivalent group that receives an alternate treatment or no treatment (control group), and random assignment to those groups with the purpose of identifying true treatment effects. This means that effects were caused by the treatment and not attributed to any outside source.

Randomization is the method wherein that which is being studied, such as a person or another unit of observation like a school or hospital, has an equal chance to be assigned to either the experimental or the control group. It attempts to ensure that no bias exists in assigning individuals to either treatment or control groups, and that the groups therefore are roughly equivalent or balanced in terms of sociodemographic or other characteristics deemed important for evaluation purposes. Such balance in the distribution of these factors in both the group receiving the intervention and the group that does not means that they probably affect the outcome in the same way. The point at which randomization occurs can vary—individuals can be randomly assigned to an intervention or control group either before or after completing a baseline assessment. With randomization, the internal validity of study findings is improved.

Even after random allocation of subjects, however, it is best to check that groups are balanced on these and all other characteristics. In other words, check to see if the random assignment was successful. Further, random assignment will not guarantee that two groups that are equivalent at the beginning of the evaluation will stay that way throughout. In other words, threats to the internal validity of the design, such as maturation and history, must still be controlled.

The value of random assignment is that it improves the evaluator's ability to infer causation to the intervention for effects observed. The effects cannot automatically be attributed to the intervention simply because participants were randomly assigned to the treatment and control groups, but the argument has been strengthened. Randomizing participants is only one part of a strong design. When the design includes randomization with the control over other threats to internal validity and a systematically implemented intervention, then causal inferences are more likely to be valid.

In the real world, the researcher will not always have the level of control needed to randomize participants. Table 5.2 provides some strategies when randomization is not ideal. A true randomized experiment cannot always be implemented in the evaluation of HIV/AIDS interventions, because these interventions may be held in settings that prohibit the use of random assignment. Having a preexisting condition may be one factor that prohibits random assignment of participants. In the study of HIV/AIDS, it would be impossible and unethical to randomly assign people into an "infected" or "noninfected" group by infecting them with the virus.

Likewise, if your intervention is implemented in an environment where potential participants are likely to interact, such as a bar, homeless shelter, or drug-free therapeutic community, the resulting threats to internal validity caused by randomization outweigh its benefits. For example, in an ecological intervention, the entire population in question participates in the intervention and is the unit of analysis. In such "whole population" studies, randomization within a setting becomes impossible. In a single setting, such as a homeless shelter, the design becomes muddied when participants are randomly assigned to either the intervention or control group. This often results in cross-over effects (also referred to as diffusion or contamination effects) where members of the experimental group communicate information with members of the control group.

In a similar vein, demoralization of the control group can occur. In this situation, the control group attempts to change on its own, almost in competition with the intervention group. Under such conditions, it becomes necessary for the evaluator to identify nonequivalent groups to compare with the treatment groups. For example, comparing the residents of a different shelter who did not receive the intervention with the residents of a shelter who did is one means of constructing a nonequivalent comparison group. In this example, all the other controls for the threats to internal validity apply as they would in a

Table 5.2. Issues and Strategies around Random Assignment of Subjects to AIDS Prevention Programs[a]

Identification and recruitment of participants	Perception that control group members are deprived of service
• One-shot needs assessment of target groups members prior to program planning and implementation (example: baseline AIDS-related KAB study of women seeking OB-GYN care) • Pipeline or case flow study of target group members over time and at the site level prior to program planning and implementation (example: ongoing monitoring and direct observation of gay/bisexual men attending an STD clinic) • Pilot study of proposed program with a small sample of subjects prior to implementation of large-scale programs (example: determine estimates of inner-city black and Hispanic women who consent to pretest counseling; HIV testing; return for posttest counseling and notification or results; and seek on-going counseling). Assessment of consent rates and attrition over time will provide realistic projections of subject flow in longitudinal preventive intervention. • Deploying outreach prevention workers to generate interest in program participation (example: using adolescent male hustlers to inform other hustlers of the AIDS prevention program). • Hiring dedicated intake workers to ensure that target group members enroll in program, follow through with program participation, and remain in the program (example: use of dedicated staff from targeted community, such as prostitutes, may maximize their program participation and reduce attrition rates).	• Provision of services to both experimental and control group member prior to random assignment of subjects (example: providing assistance with housing and other concrete needs, such as infant formula or diapers, unrelated to the AIDS educational intervention, to low-income women assigned to the control group). The service provided to the control group must be minimal to preclude it from washing out treatment effects of the intervention given to experimental group members. • Recognition of financial constraint of resources. Demands for services exceed availability of resources. • Delay preventive treatment for control group until preventive treatment is proven effective. This approach, however, may be problematic. First, if longitudinal follow-up of the experimental and control group is required, intervention cannot be offered to control group members until follow-up measurement of program participants has been completed. Second, under certain circumstances, delayed treatment would be unethical, as in the case of notification of HIV test results. • Recognition of the experimental nature of the AIDS prevention program. • Recognition that services to a limited group are better than no program service. • Provision of a minimal intervention for control group members. This approach would change a study design from "treatment–no treatment" to a "treatment–comparison group one," and hence, change the research questions and objectives being addressed.

Perception that clients' needs are critical	Misunderstanding random assignment	Objections regarding referral
• Increase participant–control group member ratio to allow more individuals to receive the AIDS prevention education intervention. The uneven distribution of individuals in the two groups requires a larger sample size and extension of program length. • Withholding a fixed number of program slots from random assignment for those perceived to need the services. The risk here is that individuals most in need of the services may be excluded from receiving the intervention because program slots are held aside; thus, excluding the truly needy may diminish detection of program effects. • Guarantee that future services will be provided to control group members.	• Remove responsibility for random assignment from AIDS prevention staff. Designate it to be the responsibility of evaluation staff. • Explain need for randomization repeatedly and in different ways, e.g., individual and group presentation. • Train others to explain the purpose of randomization (let staff market the need to their colleagues). • Hold staff meeting to discuss, negotiate, and resolve problems.	• Consider legitimacy of complaints and put them in perspective. • Randomly allocate participants by pairs (matched on ethnicity or sex, for example) to AIDS preventive intervention and control condition groups. This procedure will eliminate imbalance that will occur with random assignment of a small sample of individuals. • Have a realistic perspective of capabilities of referral agencies/organization, especially their ability to generate referrals to the AIDS prevention program. • Recognize that participant selection ratio and attrition are unknown in many service and educational programs. • Develop contingency plans. • Employ options noted in other columns of this table.

[a]Adapted from Boruch, Dennis, & Carter-Greer (1988).

randomized experimental design. Collection of baseline (pretest) data helps to ensure that the groups were equivalent at the beginning of the intervention. In other words, the evaluator creates a proxy to the randomized experiment called a *quasi-experimental design*.

In situations as outlined above, it is necessary to use designs that will enable the evaluator to arrive at interpretable results. These designs are referred to as quasi-experimental, in that the rigors of science must be adapted to the reality of the intervention settings. All of the designs discussed in this chapter could be used in situations where participants are randomly assigned to the treatment or control condition, in other words, a randomized experimental design. When randomization is contraindicated, quasi-experimental designs are applied using nonequivalent comparison groups.

CONSIDERATIONS IN USING NO-TREATMENT AND ALTERNATIVE TREATMENT GROUPS

In the following section, we discuss the various types of groups that can be used to compare with the intervention group. The basic types of groups include nontreatment groups, alternative treatment groups, and delayed treatment groups. It is important to highlight that when a randomized experimental design is implemented, the comparison group is called a control group. For quasi-experimental designs, the comparison group is a nonequivalent comparison group.

The use of a no-treatment group, a group that does not receive any treatment, strengthens the integrity of the research design, especially internal validity. At the same time, a number of issues that potentially could impinge upon the design must be addressed by the evaluator.

Choosing a Control/Comparison Condition

Building a no-treatment condition into a study design provides an unexposed group for comparison with the treatment group. The use of no-treatment groups raises an important question that all evaluators need to address: Is it ethical to deny, for the purposes of an evaluation, educational material and services that may well be effective? This is indeed a serious question, given the life-threatening nature of AIDS and high HIV seroprevalence in many areas. The flip side to this question, of course, is: How do we know the intervention is effective without the evaluation component? Too often, educators believe that any program implemented with a group should be made readily available to the public. Conversely, programs that health educators believe to be effective are offered, but not evaluated.

A viable alternative to a no-treatment condition is the use of an alternate treatment condition, which is a group of individuals who receive a different treatment than the intervention group. An alternate treatment group is one that is similar in composition to the intervention group and allows for meaningful comparison of the relative efficacy of the intervention, but maintains the integrity of the study design. This group always receives a treatment, but one that is different from the type received by the intervention group. The nature of the alternate treatment should be grounded in some theoretical rationale. Examples of alternate conditions are group-based social skills training versus a psychoeducational support group, or enhanced case management versus the usual standard of case management. If the program being evaluated is multisessioned with small-group discussion, individuals in the alternate treatment group may receive written information in the mail. If the same information is provided to members of both the treatment and alternate treatment groups, the effects of the two treatments can be compared. Example 5.1 illustrates a randomized experimental design in which a new intervention to promote safer sex practices for gay and bisexual men was evaluated against a group receiving an alternate treatment.

As can be expected in field research, established procedures cannot always be implemented as planned. While subjects in the above-noted study were randomly assigned to the two comparative treatment conditions during most of the study period, randomization was inconsistent. In one instance, the skills training program was not offered for several months. Another time, poor attendance resulted in the cancellation of the skills training intervention. Fortunately, comparison of baseline age, race, educational level, sexual practices, and HIV seroprevalence of men in the two groups revealed no systematic differences. As previously discussed, demonstrating the equivalence of group composition aids the evaluator in attributing the observed treatment effects to the intervention and not to differences in group characteristics.

One design variant is to incorporate both no-treatment and alternate treatment

---

Example 5.1. Randomized Trial with Comparison Groups Study Design

Evaluation Strategy

A group of 584 gay and bisexual men in Pittsburgh were randomized into either a skills-training intervention plus small-group lecture ($n = 319$) or a small-group lecture only ($n = 265$). The sample was recruited from the Pitt Men's Study and from the larger community of gay and bisexual men in Pittsburgh. Assessment of HIV knowledge, attitudes, and practices took place at baseline prior to the intervention and at two 6-month intervals following participation in the intervention.

Results

The evaluation showed that the skills-training plus small-group program proved to be better than the small-group-only program in one domain only. The skills-training program increased participants' use of condoms during insertive anal intercourse—from 36% of partners at the time of pretest to 80% of partners at the second follow-up. In contrast, men in the small-group-only intervention increased condom use from 44% of their partners at pretest to 55% at the second follow-up. Levels of knowledge and condom use during receptive anal intercourse between the two groups did not differ.

(SOURCE: Valdiserri *et al.*, 1989.)

groups in a study and contrast them with an experimental treatment group. This is illustrated in Example 5.2. Sometimes, even with a sound research design and a culturally competent and age-relevant intervention strategy, evaluation results can prove to be disappointing, as illustrated in Example 5.3.

Several explanations can be offered for predominantly nonsignificant findings. A ceiling effect whereby participants' scores were high at pretest could result in an intervention showing no effect in many outcome domains. Second, analysis of a sample heterogeneous by gender and race/ethnicity could attenuate effects that might appear if analyses were conducted with gender and ethnically/racially homogeneous samples. In other words, effects observed in one group may wash out or cancel the effects in another

---

Example 5.2. Study with Comparison and Control Groups Design

Evaluation Strategy

Seventy-five white and black female adolescents in a health clinic-based program were randomly assigned to one of three groups: (1) an enhanced experimental (EE) group that received an AIDS lecture plus video; (2) an experimental (E) group that received an AIDS lecture only; and (3) a control group that received no education other than a pamphlet. The use of a no-treatment control group enabled the researchers to evaluate the effects of AIDS knowledge acquired prior to the educational intervention.

All subjects completed a questionnaire that assessed knowledge about HIV transmission and condom use as well as attitudes about persons with AIDS, adoption of preventive health behaviors, and perceptions about the seriousness of AIDS. These measures were assessed after group participation only; no measures were administered prior to random assignment and group participation. An innovative method was employed to measure condom use: the distribution of prenumbered coupons that could be exchanged for free condoms at the hospital's pharmacy. The pharmacy maintained a list of numbers of the returned coupons.

Selected demographic characteristics and condom purchase behavior of participants in the three groups were initially compared to determine whether there were any systematic group differences.

Results

The two experimental AIDS education groups scored higher on the AIDS knowledge scale than the control group; the EE group was as effective as the E group. Group differences in attitudes and acquisition of condoms from the pharmacy were not statistically significant. However, among participants in the EE group who reported past purchase of condoms, a greater proportion acquired condoms. The intervention suggests that a brief intervention (E) can be effective as an enhanced intervention (EE) in increasing knowledge and reinforcing existing HIV prevention behaviors.

(SOURCE: Rickert *et al.*, 1990.)

Example 5.3. Knowledge Gains as a Function of Group Instruction

---

Evaluation Strategy

Sixty Latino and black adolescents recruited from an urban job-training program were randomly assigned to one of two experimental conditions or a control condition. Experimental group members received either: (1) a comic book, rap music verse format self-instructional guide about AIDS *with* group instruction (three 1-hour sessions), or (2) the self-instructional guide about AIDS *without* group instruction. Control group participants received information only—a fact sheet about AIDS; neither a self-instructional guide about AIDS nor group instruction about the guide was provided. Assessment focused on knowledge, attitudes, and risks related to HIV infection.

Results

Only modest support for the effectiveness of the self-instructional method was found. The adolescents assigned to the self-instructional guide plus group discussion reported that they increased the frequency of talking about AIDS with friends from pre- to posttest more than those assigned either to the self-instruction-only condition or the information-only condition. Process evaluation data indicated that participants were enthusiastic and positive about the intervention, and about one fifth reported that they wanted to learn more about AIDS and related risks.

(SOURCE: Schinke, Gordon, & Weston, 1990.)

---

group. Third, the measures used to assess the impact of the intervention may not represent what was intended. Of course, there is always the possibility that an intervention has limited impact and is truly ineffective.

Delayed Treatment or Wait-List Control/Comparison Group

In situations where a nontreatment control group is desired, one frequently used alternative is the delayed treatment or wait-list group. For example, a program could be conducted in two waves or time periods. Half of the target sample would receive the program in January and the second half 6 months later to serve as a control group for the wave-one sample.

This procedure has two drawbacks. First, the educational program is delayed for a short period of time, which raises for some the issue of denied treatment and perhaps increased psychological distress among the no-treatment group subjects. The no-treatment group cannot be given the educational treatment until the intervention and follow-up observation period is completed for the intervention group. In addition, long-term repeated follow-up assessments of the delayed treatment control group may not be feasible due to these increased delays. An application of the wait-list control group is described in Example 5.4.

Example 5.4. Study with Wait-List Control Group Design

Evaluation Strategy

A wait-list control group was used to assess the impact of stress management training on gay men's sexual behavior and immunological function. Following completion of a baseline questionnaire and venipuncture, 64 men were randomized to either a treatment or control group. After the end of an 8-week stress management training treatment cycle, both treatment and control group members completed a follow-up assessment of their sexual behavior and immunological function. Men in the wait-list control group were then offered stress management training.

(SOURCE: Coates, McKusick, Kuno, & Stites, 1989.)

MATCHING

Matching intervention and control/comparison group participants on one or more variables prior to randomization is a powerful technique for controlling the effects of unwanted variables on the experimental treatment. Selection of matching variables should be on the basis of what variables, other than those related to the experimental intervention, are most likely to affect postintervention outcome measures. For example, if a researcher believes that age, gender, or HIV status affect adoption of HIV precautionary behavior, then it might be best to remove the potential for this to occur by pairing intervention and control/comparison subjects on these three factors and randomly assigning one member of each pair to the intervention group and the other to the control/comparison group.

The intent is to improve our confidence that any effects are attributable to the intervention, rather than to differences in group characteristics of the participants. Matching ensures equivalence of intervention and control/comparison participants in terms of characteristics that are likely to affect outcome. It is important to note that with each characteristic on which you match, the more difficult it becomes to obtain a sample. If you wish to control for the three characteristics identified above, assuming two levels of HIV (positive and negative), two levels of gender (male and female), three levels of age (adult, adolescent, and pediatric), and two levels of treatment (intervention and control/comparison), you would have to identify 24 different types of participants, or 12 pairs. For example, HIV-positive/male/adult intervention group, HIV-positive/male/adult control group, and so on. If each "cell" or group contains 5 to 10 participants, a total of 120 to 240 participants will be needed to evaluate the intervention. It is best to try to identify characteristics to be matched based on some theoretical or empirical basis, before going to the expense and trouble of matching.

LONGITUDINAL VERSUS CROSS-SECTIONAL DESIGNS

In longitudinal research, data are collected over time and compared across time periods. In this design, the same group of people may be assessed over multiple time

intervention; it becomes impossible, therefore, to differentiate developmental impact from program impact.

In general, the above-noted limitations inherent in a one-group posttest-only design mean that evaluation findings must be interpreted with caution. There are too many threats to the integrity of the design to permit definitive statements about the results.

The One-Group Pretest–Posttest Design

An example of this commonly used design is shown in Fig. 5.2. A single group of subjects are assessed at baseline (O_1) and then are exposed to a treatment or program (X). Following the program, participants are assessed again (O_2). The evaluator then looks for changes between the pretest and posttest. Although those threats present in previous designs are partially alleviated by the inclusion of baseline test scores, even in this design change cannot necessarily be attributed to the program. Factors other than the program may have been responsible for the observed differences between the two groups.

Most threats to internal validity cannot be controlled in this design. Four major threats to the integrity of the one-group pretest–posttest design are: (1) history or intervening events, (2) statistical regression, (3) instrumentation, and (4) testing. First, depending on when the posttest (O_2) is administered, intervening historical events can affect the interpretation of data. It becomes impossible to determine if change was due to the program or to an outside contemporary influential event (e.g., the United States Surgeon General's national household mailing, or Magic Johnson's public disclosure of his HIV status) that occurred between the pretest and the posttest. Distribution of coupons to be exchanged for accelerated enrollment in a drug treatment program during an intervention and between assessment intervals could influence targeted outcomes as much as the intervention. Again, the use of a control group will help alleviate this problem.

A second threat involves statistical regression. In testing, when individuals have extreme baseline scores (time 1), their scores will gravitate toward the mean at follow-up

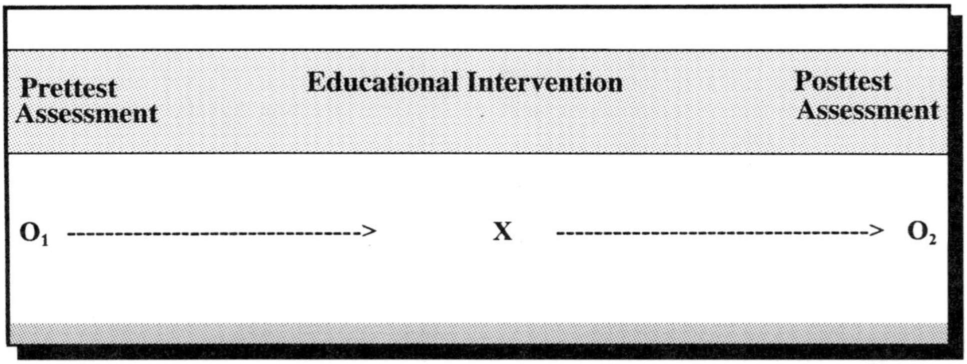

Prettest Assessment	Educational Intervention	Posttest Assessment
O_1 --------------------------->	X --------------------------------->	O_2

Figure 5.2.   The one-group pretest–posttest design. X, Intervention being tested; O, observation.

assessment (time 2). This is largely due to chance, and any changes that occur could be attributed mistakenly to the program. Two strategies will minimize this problem: (1) eliminate participants with extreme scores, and (2) use multiple measures at pretest to obtain stable baseline scores. Using an average score over time will help lessen the effects of statistical regression toward the mean.

Instrumentation, an effect that might occur if definitions of target behaviors and knowledge domains change between pretest and posttest, can be another threat to internal validity. Consistency is vital in order to make the most of comparisons between pre- and posttests. In addition, testing itself can be a catalyst to cognitive and behavioral change. Participant's preintervention attitude scores about HIV vaccine trials may influence their 6-month postintervention scores.

Interrupted Time Series Design

This is essentially a pretest–posttest design involving repeated measurement over some defined period before and after an intervention is delivered to an intervention group. With this design, a series of measurements are taken before and after the intervention. This design is often used to measure the effects of a media campaign. For example, prior to introducing a public service campaign targeted to adolescents, three knowledge–attitude–behavior surveys of adolescents' HIV-related knowledge, attitudes, and behavior conducted over a 9-month period revealed that 15% of the adolescents reported using condoms every time they had vaginal sex. Following the 1-month public service announcement (PSA) campaign, three follow-up assessments were conducted over a 9-month period. At each successive follow-up assessment, the proportion of adolescents reporting consistent condom use increased, reaching 30% at the final assessment.

The evaluator might interpret this as meaning that the campaign was effective in changing adolescents' condom use behavior. However, there is always the possibility that history or instrumentation effects could account for this increase in condom use. Further, testing effects may account for this change in condom use. The trends in the data, however, can provide some indication as to whether these threats to validity are operating. In the above example, if there were significant increases in condom use in the three assessments conducted prior to the campaign, but there was a steady increase in condom use following the campaign, then we have greater confidence that history effects were not a threat to validity. On the other hand, if the proportionate increase in condom use was the same among the three precampaign and three postcampaign assessments, the increases in condom use could not be attributed to treatment effects, i.e., to the PSA campaign. If the researcher is interested in whether the behavior is maintained over time rather than having only a transitory impact, then there must be a sufficient number of postintervention assessments to capture long-term trends.

Plotting these trends on a graph and visually inspecting them can give the evaluator insight into determining what is going on. If there is a sharp increase in condom use following the campaign, as shown in Fig. 5.3D, then inferences may be drawn about the campaign's effects.

Clearly, this was the case following Magic Johnson's public disclosure of his HIV infection and the sharp increase in the number of telephone calls to the National AIDS Hotline. Alternate sources of data, such as key informant interviews and systematic review of newspapers, can identify potential confounding events occurring close in time to the intervention (Kessler, 1993).

Designs with Control/Comparison Groups

As stated earlier, control groups refer to evaluation designs where random assignment to the intervention and nonintervention group is made. Where random assignment is not possible, a nonequivalent comparison group is constructed (Cook & Campbell, 1979). This is the primary differentiation between the randomized experimental design and the quasi-experimental design. As such, the two types of designs will be discussed together.

Posttest-Only Design with Nonequivalent Groups

The schematic of this design is presented in Fig. 5.4. Group A receives a treatment (X) with a posttest observation (O_1), while group B receives the posttest only (O_2). This is an example of a quasi-experimental design. The latter group is called the no-treatment group or comparison group. Comparison group members should be as similar (e.g., demographically) as possible to intervention group members, even though they do not receive the preventive intervention. Neither group is tested prior to the intervention in this design. Inferences about the impact of the intervention are based on the comparison between the intervention group and the comparison group scores at O_2.

A major shortcoming with this design is the lack of preintervention assessment on either group on scales similar to or the same as the posttest assessment. As Cook and Campbell (1979) point out, archival data may be used to establish baseline assessments. Therefore, the extent of change in the experimental group cannot be assessed. Any changes in posttest measures may be attributable to differences in group characteristics, rather than the intervention. Moreover, given the lack of random assignment, we cannot be sure that the two groups were equivalent before implementation of the intervention. A variant of the nonequivalent control group design is described in Example 5.7.

The inclusion of a control group minimizes effects due to historical events or maturational trends. The absence of baseline data makes it impossible to assess change. Also, we cannot ascertain if differences between the treatment and control groups are due to the educational treatment or preexisting differences between the groups ("selection bias"). Because, even when randomly assigned, the two groups' knowledge of HIV infection and their perceptions of risk behaviors are uncertain prior to the educational treatment; therefore, the information obtained cannot be interpreted as program effects.

The No-Treatment Group Design with Pretest and Posttest

This design has great applicability to the community-based organizations (CBO) and AIDS service organizations (ASO) and often leads to interpretable results. It is a powerful design in terms of controlling for threats to internal validity. Typically,

A. Steady increase before and after the intervention.

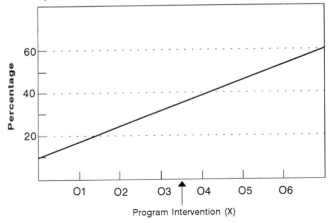

B. Regular cyclical changes before and after the intervention.

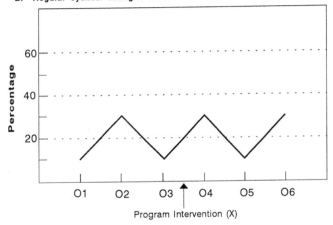

Figure 5.3. Four potential outcomes from a hypothetical study design.

participants are randomly assigned to a group exposed to the intervention or to a no-treatment control group. This design is diagramed in Fig. 5.5.

In this design, the treatment group is pretested (O_{1A}) and receives an educational intervention (X). Following the intervention, participants are given a posttest (O_{2A}) or readministration of the pretest. The pretest and posttest are simultaneously administered to both the treatment and control groups. The only difference between the groups is that the second group, O_{1B}, receives no treatment, and thus serves as a control group. Ideally, the control group's characteristics will be similar to those of intervention group members due to randomization. In this design, effects are attributed to the intervention when two conditions are met: (1) changes in the intervention group are in the predicted direction

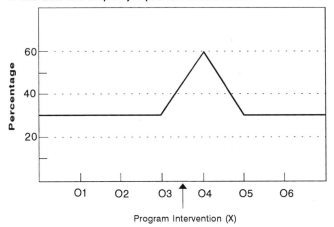

C. Immediate and temporary impact of the intervention.

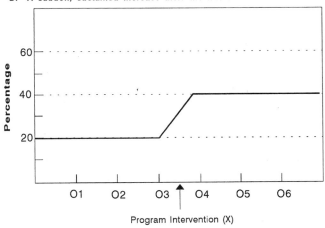

D. A sudden, sustained increase after the intervention.

Figure 5.3. (*Continued*)

	Educational Intervention	Test Assessment
Group A	X--->	O_1
Group B		O_2

Figure 5.4. Posttest-only design with nonequivalent groups. X, Intervention being tested; O, observation.

Example 5.7.   Variation of the Nonequivalent Control Group Design

---

Evaluation Strategy

A nonequivalent control group was used in evaluating a single, one-to-one AIDS educational session with 662 IDUs in Cleveland recruited from the street and a methadone maintenance program. After having completed a personal interview that assessed AIDS knowledge and risk behaviors and, subsequently, the intervention, participants were contacted 3 months later and reinterviewed. About half of the sample ($n = 338$) completed both the pre- and posttest.

Results

There were no systematic differences between IDUs who completed both the pre- and posttest and those who completed the pretest only. Since 71.4% of the IDUs were recruited from the streets, the "3-month" follow-up interview was administered between 36 to 448 days after the intervention. Thus, treating the pretest sample as nonequivalent controls for the follow-up sample of respondents who were interviewed during the same time period enabled the researchers to maximize the follow-up rate.

Impact evaluation indicated that increased knowledge was related to safer injection practices. When the length of time between the intervention and the posttest was controlled, there were no significant differences between groups. Thus, the knowledge differences between the experimental and comparison groups cannot be attributed definitively to the intervention.

(SOURCE: Feucht, Stephens, & Gibbs, 1991.)

---

from pretest to posttest; and (2) the intervention group's scores at posttest will be greater than the control group's scores, in the predicted direction.

With random assignment of subjects, this design controls for most of the threats to the integrity of evaluation. The two groups are assumed to be similar prior to treatment. There are still four situations, however, which could potentially threaten the results.

	Pretest Assessment	Educational Intervention	Posttest Assessment
R	O_{1A} ---------------------------------->	X ------------------------->	O_{2A}
	O_{1B}		O_{2B}

Figure 5.5.   The untreated control group design with pretest and posttest. X, Intervention being tested; O, observation; R, randomization.

The first uncontrolled threat is that of selection maturation, which occurs when one group is growing or changing at a rate faster than the other group, and the growth is unrelated to the intervention. For example, if you survey two groups at pretest and expose only group 1 to an AIDS prevention program, you would expect to see differences between them at posttest and predict that group 1 would have a higher level of knowledge and greater behavioral change than group 2. Ideally, these differences would be attributed to the educational treatment.

The researcher, however, must be able to rule out any possibility that the differences originated in the treatment group are due to their being more informed at pretest, are brighter, or have a greater aptitude for learning than the control group. This can be done by establishing, through a *t*-test or analysis of variance, whether the two groups proved to be equal on selected characteristics at pretest.

A second situation suggesting the presence of maturational trends occurs when scores for the treatment group improve and those for the control group remain unchanged over time. Typically, all groups will demonstrate some change over time. The scores from observation to observation will not be identical. Consequently, it is essential to account for the lack of change. In the absence of a reasonable explanation, results must be examined and interpreted with caution.

A second threat to the internal validity of the evaluation is the presence of effects due to instrumentation, i.e., problems indigenous to questionnaires and surveys that increase the disparity between the treatment and control groups at pretest. This problem may emerge if the pre- and posttest versions of the instrument are not the same. Changing the instrument may produce effects that are independent of the intervention effects.

When the situation precludes the random assignment of participants to the intervention and no-intervention group, a nonequivalent comparison group can be used in place of the control group. For example, if the intervention was a school-based program, the evaluator may identify school A as the intervention site and school B as the comparison site. This would be necessary to eliminate diffusion or cross-over effects and the disillusioned control group effect, which are threats to the internal validity of the evaluation.

The use of the quasi-experimental design carries with it additional threats to the internal validity of the evaluation that normally would be controlled for by randomization. One threat associated with the use of the comparison group is an instrumentation-related issue. It is important to view the initial frequencies (the proportion of respondents in each response category of a particular question) for each group and to look for situations where data are clustered at the low end (floor effects) or high end (ceiling effects) of the scale. This is particularly problematic when floor or ceiling effects appear in one group and not in the other. If such effects are noted, it may be necessary to rescale the items or regroup the samples in a meaningful way.

A third threat to the integrity of the evaluation is called differential statistical regression. (As discussed earlier in this section, statistical regression occurs when an individual or group scores extremely high or low at time 1 and their scores move toward the mean at time 2.) When statistical regression affects one group and not the other, then it is differential. This occurs when comparison groups are drawn from populations different from those receiving the treatment. If you were to implement a treatment group in an area where the average level of AIDS-related knowledge is low and a comparison group from a population where the average AIDS-related knowledge level is high, you might select participants for the latter by matching their scores with those of the former. At face value, this would seem to be a good idea. However, low scorers do not accurately represent a population and will, by statistical regression, show an increase in scores at posttest. Typically, such differentials yield findings that indicate the control group performed better at pretest than did the treatment group.

Finally, local history (the interaction between participants and historical events) can interfere with the interpretability of results. For example, in evaluating an AIDS education program in a gay bar, a second bar could serve as the comparison group. The characteristics of each could impact the integrity of the evaluation. If patrons in one bar were raucous, if the bar was poorly lighted, and if it served complimentary drinks to patrons, and then its patrons were exposed to the program later in the evening than in the other bar, differential results (independent of the program) could occur. To avoid such situations, it is important to visit and choose program sites that are as comparable, or neutral, as possible.

Solomon Four-Group Design

This design, shown in Table 5.3, is superior to the randomized pretest–posttest control group design because it removes one potential threat to external validity—test reactivity. Two groups are added to the design that do not receive the pretest observation. One of these groups receives the intervention and one does not. This configuration enables the evaluator to control for test reactivity or testing effects. Following completion of the experimental intervention, all groups are assessed. With randomization, one can assume that the pretest scores of the two groups at T_1 would be similar to the scores of the nonintervention group and the no-test group at T_3 who were pretested at this time. In the absence of the pretest, the potential for an interaction between pretest scores and the intervention are removed. This design requires a large number of subjects and is labor-intensive in terms of program delivery and measurement efforts. Example 5.8 describes a

Table 5.3. Randomized Solomon Four-Group Design

	Time[a]		
Group	T1 Pretest	T2 Treatment	T3 Posttest
Pretested	O_1	X_1	O_2
Pretested	O_3		O_4
Not pretested		X_2	O_5
Not pretested			O_6

[a]X, intervention being tested; O, observation; R, randomization.

In terms of real-world significance, however, the evaluator needs to know how well the program achieved its goals of safer sex practice. By their own report, participants are still exposing themselves and others to HIV infection. Essentially, when the desired outcome is consistently protected vaginal or anal intercourse, anything short of 100% condom use can be construed as program failure. From the perspective of HIV transmission, such failure takes on added meaning, especially in communities with high HIV seroprevalence. Thus, programmatically significant effects of sufficient magnitude can be as important, if not more so, than statistically significant effects.

Effect size refers to a standardized unit of change in one group or a difference in changes between two groups; it assesses the magnitude of these changes (Kazis, Anderson, & Meenan, 1989). It serves as a criterion for setting the level of power of an intervention.

Conceptually, effect size can be determined a priori by ascertaining the differences in mean knowledge or attitudinal scores or in risk behaviors among members of the intervention and control groups that will be considered substantively significant. For example, a 20% difference in condom use immediately following participation in an AIDS education program and 30% difference between groups 6 months later can serve as the criteria to gauge the effectiveness of this program. From a practical standpoint, the significance of this gain and the value of mean differences between groups need to be determined. Statistical methods are required, however, to determine the magnitude of the effect (i.e., the proportion of variance accounted for) in outcomes. Unfortunately, effect size varies according to the nature of the sample and adherence to a standardized program protocol (Sechrest & Yeaton, 1981). As such, the obtained effect size is bound to the sample on which it was calculated and the time of testing. Increases in the integrity of the sampling procedure and strict adherence to the study protocol should increase the observed effect size.

Hence, it is important to establish realistic and meaningful benchmarks by which to assess program success in the sometimes nebulous areas of behavioral, attitudinal, and knowledge-related change data. One alternative is to look at the data from other research studies and do normative-like comparisons between your outcomes and those of other researchers (Sechrest & Yeaton, 1981; Fitz-Gibbon & Morris, 1987). Amounts of change previously experienced as a result of interventions can become criteria against which you assess your success.

Evaluators and educators can also rate what kind of and how much change they would expect to see in participants at the end of an intervention and at specified intervals thereafter (Sechrest et al., 1982, 1983). The strength of treatment effects should be considered within the context of the theoretical rationale for intended effects and the clinical significance of effects.

Unintended program effects should be monitored as part of the evaluation process. Sometimes these effects are desirable, but they can also be detrimental to participants (Sechrest et al., 1982, 1983). An AIDS prevention program that directs women to be assertive with sexual partners and encourages them to use condoms, for example, may unintentionally provoke their partners to engage in domestic violence.

Program evaluators may be concerned if evaluation findings indicate that a program had little or no effects, or if there were inconsistent differences with regard to the direction of program effects. AIDS educators new to the field of evaluation should be comforted by the fact that many evaluations show ambiguous program effects. While statistical hypotheses are conventionally stated in the form of null hypotheses—that there are no program effects—program personnel, for fear their funding and agency backing will be terminated, are often reluctant to disclose such nonsignificant results. Articles in professional journals are biased as well in that editorial boards tend to limit the publication of studies that show no program effects.

However, evaluation studies are not only bottom-line declarations of absolute success or failure of an intervention. The resultant studies identify valuable "secondary" information, such as client characteristics. The process of the evaluation can identify program implementation problems that might be correctable. Further statistical analysis of the components of the intervention may identify what aspects of the program are most promising and candidates for more intensive development. In general, the results of an evaluation are more than a "thumbs up or down" to a program. The information can provide the agency with a plethora of information for programmatic and policy-oriented decision-making.

Secular trends can hinder researchers' ability to detect statistically significant intervention effects (Leviton & Valdiserri, 1990). Program-related change effects can be obscured because of either floor or ceiling effects (Sechrest et al., 1982, 1983). Floor effects occur when the pretest is insensitive to difference among participants, making it difficult to assess differential change. Ceiling effects make it difficult to discriminate among participants following a program because, prior to their participation, they had already made significant reductions in their high-risk sexual and drug use practices (see Example 5.10). Even slight reductions in high-risk behaviors may be washed out because of ceiling effects. These changes may be attributed to several factors, including fear of becoming infected with HIV or switching from injecting heroin to smoking crack or snorting cocaine.

Thus, in a controlled design, both floor and ceiling effects might lead the evaluator to conclude that no differences existed between the group who received the preventive intervention and the group receiving a different (or no) intervention. Longer-term follow-up assessments may show differences between groups. When participants are given no room for improvement, however (e.g., consistent condom use at the onset and in all sexual encounters over the course of a program), postprogram changes may not be detected.

If an evaluation shows no differences among subjects following their participation in an AIDS preventive intervention, several checks are in order. The programs should be scrutinized for possible methodological flaws. These include nonequivalent control groups, lack of random allocation of subjects to experimental and control conditions, inappropriate statistical analyses, unreliable measures, small sample size, and ceiling effects in knowledge and attitudinal and behavioral changes (Sechrest & Yeaton, 1981). If a program evaluation results in a true, no-difference finding, disclosure of such information might save other evaluators the trouble of replicating a program's shortcomings. Even when the results of a program evaluation show little or no effects, an agency may opt to retain the program because of its emotional commitment, community good will, or lack of harm to participants.

Example 5.10. Ceiling Effects in a Study of Gay Men in New Zealand

---

Evaluation Strategy

One hundred fifty-nine gay men in New Zealand were recruited through gay venues and randomly assigned to one of four experimental treatment conditions—a video, individual HIV counseling, an eroticization of safer-sex group, or a safer-sex guidelines group—or a control condition. All men were assessed at baseline, prior to the intervention, and 6 months following the intervention. The control group received assessment only.

Results

Evaluation of the intervention revealed the presence of a ceiling effect. Prior to the intervention, 75% of the sample reported practicing safer sex and at follow-up the proportion increased slightly, to 82%. No significant differences were detected at the $P < 0.05$ level across the intervention and control groups. When the P value was raised to < 0.10, which the researchers considered to represent a significant trend, the HIV-counseling group appeared to be more effective in terms of an increased number of men adopting safer sex. The eroticization of safer sex group showed a trend of greater avoidance of anal intercourse compared to the other treatment and control conditions.

(SOURCE: Robert & Rosser, 1990.)

Statistical Power

The power of an intervention or experiment refers to the quantitative description of its sensitivity to the presence of change or to differences that can be termed statistically significant (Keppel, 1973). The power of an intervention is important in the planning and interpretation of a study.

The evaluator is often faced with the difficult task of determining the effect size before a study begins. Power analysis enables the evaluator to estimate the effect size. Rather than stating that there will be significant results, the researcher is expected to predict the magnitude of effects between the treatment and control/comparison groups.

Linked to estimates of effect size is the calculation of minimum sample size. Power analysis allows for the determination of the minimum sample size needed in order to obtain the estimated effect size. Without estimates of sample size, a statistically nonsignificant finding may be interpreted to mean that the intervention had no effect when, in fact, a larger sample might have produced the desired effects. Only when it can be demonstrated that the sample size was adequate can a nonsignificant result be interpretable (Moher, Dulberg, & Wells, 1994). Hence, power is critical for interpreting results of an intervention, and explaining a weak effect size or nonsignificant findings.

The power of any given statistical test refers to the probability of rejecting the null hypothesis (i.e., no differences). In statistical terms, power = $1 - \beta$, the region under the normal curve where one can safely reject the null hypothesis with minimal chance for error. It is dependent on several interrelated criteria (Keppel, 1973; Cohen & Cohen, 1975):

- The region of rejection of the null hypothesis when an alternative hypothesis is true, and the size of the level of significance, i.e., alpha level, and whether the test is one-tailed or two-tailed; thus, the probability of making a correct decision when the null hypothesis is false (power increases as alpha increases).
- The size of the sample (power increases with increasing sample size).
- Treatment effects, or the magnitude of the effect size (power increases with increasing effect size).
- Uncontrolled sources of variance (power increases with a reduction in uncontrolled variance).
- Unbiased estimates of parameters of interest (power increases with the reduction of bias).

There are no standardized criteria for setting a level of power. Often, power is driven by the size of the sample available to the researcher and the significance level. Statistically, the larger the sample, the greater one's chances of detecting statistically significant results (rejecting the null hypothesis). Ethically, the evaluator needs to estimate the minimum sample size needed for the desired effect size. This way, as few people as possible will be subjected to the untested intervention. Further, if it can be demonstrated, a priori, that the intervention will not have an effect on the available sample size, resources would not be wasted. The authors refer the reader to Cohen (1988) for a more detailed discussion of power analysis.

CONCLUSION

In the era of AIDS, no one lives in a vacuum. Virtually everyone has the opportunity to be exposed to AIDS-related information, from the media, in schools, on the streets, and on public transportation systems. Hence, the effectiveness of any new intervention must be viewed in light of preexisting information—some of which is systematically and some randomly obtained—prior to delivery of an HIV prevention program. To identify program effects correctly, a sound study design is needed at the program development stage. As discussed, selecting a study design is not just a matter of scientific and technical issues, but it also entails attention to substantive, ethical, and practical issues. This includes decisions regarding the use of experimental versus quasi-experimental designs, the use of no-treatment control/comparison groups, and the ethics associated with random assignments and the delay of treatment.

In effect, the evaluator is forced to balance the threats to the internal validity of the evaluation against the barriers to implementing a more rigorous evaluation design. There is little value in identifying an evaluation design that will be unacceptable to the community for whom it will be implemented. Consequently, it may be necessary to sacrifice some rigor to obtain timely information that can help in decision-making. Community involvement in these decisions is essential for the acceptance of the intervention (see Chapter 3).

6

Quantitative Measures in Evaluation

This chapter reviews how one constructs quantitative measures to assess knowledge, attitudes, behaviors, and intentions associated with HIV/AIDS and how these measures can be used to evaluate an intervention. Specifically, it focuses on ways to ensure confidence in the evaluation results.

QUANTITATIVE ASSESSMENT

Whether in grade school, secondary school, or in college, everyone has taken some form of a test. In any testing situation, a domain—the area of assessment to be tested—is defined. In a test of basic mathematics, the domain would include assessing the student's ability to add, subtract, multiply, and divide. With respect to AIDS, the various domains might include the spectrum of HIV infection, modes of transmission, beliefs about personal risk and efficacy of treatment for HIV, sexual and drug practices, sexual risk reduction, drug-related risk reduction, and HIV symptoms.

Quantitative assessment is based on numeric responses. Variables such as number of sexual contacts, the degree to which you believe that condoms prevent HIV transmission, and proportion of correct answers on a knowledge test are all examples of quantitative data.

DATA COLLECTION TOOLS

Various methods can be used for the quantitative assessment of knowledge, attitudes, beliefs, and intentions. Assessment of these domains is usually conducted by means of a survey, which could be by mail, telephone, or face-to-face. Structured and semistructured interviews, checklists, performance measures, diaries, chart reviews, self-administered questionnaires, and idiographic measures are seven primary data collection strategies that can be employed for quantitative assessment. When personnel and funds are adequate, interviews are generally preferable to self-administered questionnaires. Data are collected by a trained interviewer. Interviewers can probe and clarify participants' responses and note subtleties in responses that might not be detected in pencil-and-paper inventories. Self-administered questionnaires are inappropriate to use with populations that have poor reading skills or who are illiterate.

Structured Interviews

Structured interviews have predetermined, standardized questions, with the range of responses typically precoded to facilitate the transfer of data to the computer. This ensures that all questions are worded in the same way and are in the same sequence. An interviewer ensures not only that participants understand all the questions, but he or she also provides a human connection with the participants.

There is always some chance that participants may be threatened by interviewers, especially if detailed sexual and drug-related histories are taken. Under such circumstances, the validity of participant responses may be questionable. Respondents may choose to withhold information or give socially desirable responses to please an interviewer.

Semistructured Interviews

Semistructured interviews combine structured questions and responses with open-ended questions in which responses vary from participant to participant. This format allows for the standardized collection of a core (and therefore, easily quantifiable) of variables and a greater latitude in participants' responses. Precoded response categories are used, when necessary, to elicit responses from subjects.

Space should be reserved to record responses that do not fit into the given categories (hence, the need for an "other" category) and also for more detailed qualitative comments. In-depth analysis of response patterns allows for insights into participants' attitudes and values, as well as some of the reasons for their behaviors.

Probed or Prompted Responses

Sometimes study respondents are unable to answer an open-ended question. Rather than facing the risk of obtaining a "don't know" response or "no" answer, the interviewer can provide a list of possible responses when respondents are unable to mention any on their own. The layout of the interview form can be designed to note differences between probed and unprobed responses. The use of structured probes is shown in Example 6.1.

Prompted responses to questions—questions that cue a response—rely more heavily on the respondent's ability to recognize rather than recall a method or practice. One example that illustrates this point is an item asking about the use of various types of birth control. When a sample of women receiving hospital-based OB/GYN services were asked what kinds of birth control methods they had ever used and the interviewer did not read a list of methods, 6% reported they practiced anal intercourse (Mantell & DiVittis, 1990). When a different sample attending the same women's health clinics was prompted by specifically asking about the use of anal intercourse as a birth control method, 12.6% responded in the affirmative (DiVittis et al., 1990a).

Prompting is especially important when a researcher has reason to believe that respondents will give a socially desirable response and underreport a behavior. Differential responses in relation to prompted and unprompted items, however, may also be

---

Example 6.1.   Structured Probes for a Structured Interview

An interviewer might ask a subject the following question: "Why don't you (always) use birth control?" The respondent would be expected to answer this open-ended question from his or her personal perspective. First, the interviewer will record all responses given by the respondent. For each structured probe that is spontaneously mentioned by the respondent, the interviewer would check the box next to respondent-generated. This includes recording all spontaneous responses that are not listed as one of the structured probes. These responses would be recorded in the respondent's words under the Other category. However, if the respondent hesitates, does not know what to say, or does not mention one of the structured probes, the interviewer will prompt the respondent by reading the possible responses (probes). The interviewer would then check the box next to interviewer-prompted, and circle the appropriate response.

- Too costly/can't afford   [ ] Respondent-generated   [ ] Interviewer-prompted

Yes	No	Nonapplicable	Don't know/unsure	Refuses
1	2	7	8	9

- Don't need it (for   [ ] Respondent-generated   [ ] Interviewer-prompted
  example, sterile,
  vasectomy, past
  menopause)

Yes	No	Nonapplicable	Don't know/unsure	Refuses
1	2	7	8	9

- Wants a pregnancy   [ ] Respondent-generated   [ ] Interviewer-prompted

Yes	No	Nonapplicable	Don't know/unsure	Refuses
1	2	7	8	9

- Partner dislikes,   [ ] Respondent-generated   [ ] Interviewer-prompted
  doesn't believe in

Yes	No	Nonapplicable	Don't know/unsure	Refuses
1	2	7	8	9

- Other (specify)   [ ] Respondent-generated   [ ] Interviewer-prompted
  _____

Yes	No	Nonapplicable	Don't know/unsure	Refuses
1	2	7	8	9

(SOURCE: Adapted from National Institute on Drug Abuse, Community Research Branch, 1988.)

attributed to knowledge differences. For example, with respect to birth control, inability to name a method spontaneously may be attributed to either superficial or a lack of technical knowledge about a method (McGinn, Bamba, & Balma, 1989).

When conducting structured or semistructured interviews, the use of "cue," "show," or "flash" cards (precoded response cards that are given to respondents) may be helpful for certain questions. Table 6.1 provides an illustration of a cue card for a question about frequency of vaginal sex. If an evaluator or AIDS educator believes that subjects will have difficulty remembering the response choices, it is a good idea to hand them one of these cards when the question is asked. Cue cards can be of great use in answering questions regarding sensitive issues (e.g., income level), rather than forcing subjects to verbalize answers they would rather not make public. Respondents can point to the letter or number beside the response that most accurately describes their situation. Cue cards also serve as a prop, putting some respondents at ease during an interview.

Sometimes it is helpful to display response choices on a cue card in picture as well as in written form, especially when respondents have low literacy or may be unfamiliar with the written word. Familiarity with the names of various birth control methods is one such example. A pictorial cue card of birth control devices is shown in Fig. 6.1.

Checklists

A checklist is a respondent-based, self-reported, data collection tool. The respondent is presented with a series of events and asked to indicate whether he or she has experienced the event within an identified period of time. This type of assessment has been most commonly used to identify significant life events. For example, questions such as, "Have any relatives been seriously injured in the past 6 months?" are presented to each respondent. Respondents indicate "yes" or "no" to each item. This tool is said to be respondent-based in that each individual self-defines what is being requested. In the above example, the respondent decides who is a relative and what a serious injury entails. Checklists can be incorporated into interviews, which in turn vary in how structured they are.

Similar applications of behavioral events can be applied in the evaluation of HIV/AIDS prevention programs. For example, checklist items such as, "Have you practiced unsafe sex in the past six months?" allow the respondent to define the meaning of unsafe sex. In this case, the interviewer probes for precise meaning to each aspect of the events

Table 6.1. Cue Card
with Frequency Responses

Card G
Every day
Several times a week (but not every day)
1–2 times a week
1–2 times a month
Never, none of the time

Example 6.2. Goal Attainment Scale

As part of *Night School*, an HIV prevention education program for gay and bisexual men, participants constructed and completed a goal attainment scale (GAS). A blank GAS sheet with the headings: sexual behavior, drug behavior, health behavior, and two with other (see below) was given to participants. Participants were instructed to identify at least one behavior they desired to change. At the zero point, they were to identify how they behaved currently. At each extreme, participants were to indicate the best possible outcome (+2) and the worst outcome (−2) they could expect in 6 months. After 6 months, they were asked to rate where they stood. Positive movement across the group would be seen as program success.

Sexual Behavior	Drug Behavior	Health Behavior	Other	Other
Condom use during anal sex				
+2 Use condoms each time have anal sex				
+1				
0 Use condoms with new partners, not with current.				
−1				
−2 Stop using condoms with casual partners as well				

(SOURCE: Mantell *et al.*, 1989.)

Example 6.3.   Idiographic Assessment of Life Goals

- First, for you to have the most satisfying life possible, what are the main things you want to accomplish?
- Now, for you to have the most satisfying life possible, what problems facing you do you want to solve?
- Now, for you to have the most satisfying life possible, what things do you want to prevent or avoid?
- Now, for you to have the most satisfying life possible, what things do you want to keep pretty much the same as they are now?
- Now, for you to have the most satisfying life possible, what commitments do you want to let go of? ("Commitments" can mean "responsibilities" or "things that other people want or expect you to do.")
- Of all the goals you've just told me about, are there any that you haven't been able to do anything about in the past month because your health got in the way?

For each of the first five questions, participants were also asked:

- What important things have you been doing over the last month to reach these goals?

   Of these, what *three* activities matter most in reaching these goals?

(SOURCE: Rapkin, & Smith, 1992. Reproduced with permission.)

   The use of computer-assisted interviewing has some definite advantages. The cost-benefit of immediate data input and error-free questioning increases the accuracy of the data collection process. Further, by providing a private space where the respondent is not speaking to a person (as in the case of ACASI), there is greater likelihood that participants will respond honestly. The imposition of a computer between the interviewer and the respondent (as in the case of CAPI) may be viewed by some as distancing. However, it may be no more disruptive than having the interviewer write everything the respondent says on paper.

   The major drawbacks to computer-assisted interviewing in program evaluation include cost and training. First, the basic hardware and software development necessary for this type of interviewing may drain the resources of many agencies. Second, as in the case of ACASI, it presupposes familiarity with the use of computers. In the absence of such familiarity, training time before the onset of the interview will be required.

FORMAT OF QUESTIONS

   In designing appropriate items, health educators and program evaluators need to consider not only how they will collect the data and the domains to be investigated, but the response format. Various types of question structure and response categories are available: (1) true–false, (2) multiple-choice tests, (3) fill in the blanks, (4) Likert-type scales, (5) physiological indicators, and (6) frequency indicators.

True–False

True–false tests typically measure knowledge. A declarative statement is presented to participants who are forced to determine if the statement is true or false. For example, the statement, "HIV can be transmitted by sharing food and utensils," illustrates a true–false item concerned with mode of HIV transmission. Sometimes a third response category of "unsure" is included and is, functionally, an incorrect answer, as shown in Example 6.4. Correct (true) responses are coded as 1 and incorrect (false) responses as 0. "Don't know" responses often have their own code and may be analyzed separately or recoded and treated as an incorrect response. Knowledge indices are obtained by determining the sum of correct responses or by taking a mean (average) across all items. When taking a mean, a perfect score is 1.0 and the worst possible score is 0.0. Such tests are easily administered and result in scores applicable to most standard statistical analyses. In addition, these tests are easily scored and lend themselves to computer analyses.

There are, nonetheless, several disadvantages. If the same test is given to the same participants at different times, there is the possibility that participants will have learned the correct answers from the initial test (i.e., test reactivity). In this case, gains made at the second testing would not be due to the intervention. The test also requires literate participants, and there is always a chance they might obtain correct answers by guess-work.

Multiple-Choice Tests

Multiple-choice tests are those in which an incomplete statement, or item root, is presented and the respondent selects from three or four responses that would best complete it. Example 6.5 illustrates a multiple-choice item that assesses participants' level of knowledge about the HIV epidemic.

Multiple-choice tests require that participants recognize the correct answer rather than recall it. Generally, most people possess better recognition than recall, which helps to increase their chances of answering a question correctly, thereby maximizing total scores on a knowledge scale. (Again, the danger exists for guessing correct answers.) As with true–false tests, multiple-choice tests are easily administered, easily scored, and

---

Example 6.4. Sample True–False Item

A person who is infected with HIV can look and feel healthy and well.

     True   False   Don't Know/Unsure

Example 6.5. Sample Multiple Choice Item

The number of women diagnosed with AIDS in the United States in 1994 was approximately:

   a. 5,000   b. 10,000   c. 14,000   d. 35,000   e. 50,000   f. 75,000

---

readily available for computer analysis. Yet, multiple-choice items are more difficult to construct than true–false items. Each possible response should appear equally correct to the uninformed respondent. As such, it is often difficult to construct reasonable incorrect responses.

Fill in the Blanks

Fill-ins are items where a key word or phrase is left out and the respondent is required to fill in the blank to complete the statement correctly. Example 6.6 illustrates a fill-in-the-blank-type item. In this example, the participant should write the word "anonymous" in the blank to complete the item. The advantages are the same as those for true–false and multiple-choice formats. Likewise, the same disadvantages apply. Yet, fill-ins are generally more difficult and require that participants recall rather than recognize the correct response. It can also be difficult to generate items for which a single correct response applies. This ambiguity may not only confuse the participant but cause scoring problems for evaluators.

Likert-Type Scales

Many quantitative attitudinal (and some behavioral) measures use Likert-type scales. This scaling method has a set of intervals assumed to be equal, with extremes anchored by opposites (strongly agree/strongly disagree). Table 6.4 presents three examples of Likert-type scales.

In Table 6.4A, the center point provides the participant with a neutral response. (The center of any odd-interval Likert-type scale is a noncommittal response and generally labeled "unsure" or "don't know.") Many researchers consider this "dead" information, as the participant has not committed to either the positive or negative side of the scale. Instead, they recommend the use of even-interval scales, such as in Table 6.4B and C, in which the respondent is forced to choose one side of the scale.

Example 6.6. Sample Fill-In Item

_____ HIV testing means that a person's name never gets used when recording his or her test results.

Table 6.4. Examples of Three Forms of Likert-Type Scales

A. Odd-numbered scale, all intervals labeled

Disagree	Somewhat disagree	Unsure	Somewhat agree	Agree
1	2	3	4	5

B. Even-numbered scale, all intervals labeled

Strongly disagree	Disagree	Somewhat disagree	Somewhat agree	Agree	Strongly agree
1	2	3	4	5	6

C. Even-numbered scale, only extremes labeled

Strongly disagree					Strongly agree
1	2	3	4	5	6

The difference between Table 6.4B and C is that the middle intervals in B are individually labeled. This can be both a boon and a hindrance to the participant. Depending on the number of middle items, it is sometimes difficult to derive meaningful labels for each. In those instances, it is helpful to identify the anchors and allow participants to choose their own distance from the extremes.

There are many advantages to using Likert-type scale items. First, scales are easily and inexpensively administered. Second, they are easy to quantify and construct as scaled data. By this we mean that the numbers generated from this scale fit into parametric statistical analysis (e.g., t-tests, analysis of variance, and regression analysis). Last, they can be administered pre- and postintervention to measure changes in HIV-related knowledge, attitudes, and behaviors.

Several limitations are apparent. First, because of the wording of these statements, participants may respond in ways that seem appropriate or socially desirable rather than according to their actual feelings. Second, reactivity to attitudinal testing may occur; simply raising certain issues may lead to attitudinal change. Third, the labels attached to response choices may be confusing to some participants. For example, if the intervals include strongly agree, agree, somewhat agree, somewhat disagree, disagree, and strongly disagree, participants may find it difficult to differentiate between the middle categories of somewhat disagree and somewhat agree. Finally, response set may occur. This means that the respondent may fall into a pattern of responses (i.e., all strongly agree or strongly disagree), rather than reading each individual item and responding to it, independent of the surrounding items.

One means to test for response sets is to include two versions of an item and word them in different directions so that consistency in responding would require the respondent to agree with one item and disagree with the second. For example, including the items, "AIDS is a major health problem among African-American women" and "AIDS has had little impact on African-American women," requires the participant to answer in opposite directions if he or she is answering the item consistently. If the participant agrees with the first statement, he/she should disagree with the second statement.

Physiological Indicators

Physiological indicators are most frequently used to assess three areas in HIV-related studies: abstinence from drugs, HIV seroconversion, and the presence of an STD. Through repeated urine analyses, the evaluator can determine a person's compliance with abstinence from injecting, popping, snorting, or smoking drugs. Depending on the number of days elapsed since last drug use, if the urine is clean, compliance would be assumed. For the participant who is seronegative on entering the program, serostatus (as determined by repeated HIV testing) would be a criterion measure reflecting the practice of safer sex and injection behaviors and/or related risk reduction. These physiological measures provide relatively accurate and reliable information and serve as a validation technique when used in combination with self-report questionnaires.

There are several disadvantages to using physiological measures. The process is time-consuming. Depending on the laboratory used, participants may have to wait several weeks to learn their HIV status. Use of laboratory resources is also labor-intensive. If, for example, HIV test results are used as an outcome measure, some staff will need intensive training in pre- and posttest counseling, as well as sufficient time in which to counsel participants. Further, HIV test results themselves are not 100% accurate. As with any test, specificity (ability of a test to detect correctly individuals who are not HIV-infected) and sensitivity (ability of a test to detect correctly individuals who are HIV-infected) must be taken into account. Given that the tests only yield the outcome, or bottom line, they provide an incomplete picture. We cannot learn anything about the process of the behavioral change from laboratory test results. In addition, the tests are time-bound. A negative urine toxicology test to cocaine use means that the person was "clean" at least 1 week prior to testing (the average time for cocaine to metabolize from the system). Finally, the ethics of the situation must be considered, with participants' rights paramount at all times.

Frequency Indicators

Frequency indicators are used to assess how often a behavior occurs. The most common use of frequency indicators in HIV prevention is in the assessment of sexual behavior and substance use. Three methods are typically used: frequency counts, Likert-type scales, and proportions. An example in relation to sexual behavior (insertive anal intercourse over a period of 2 months) is shown in Table 6.5.

The goal is the same for each method: estimating the frequency with which the participant used a condom during insertive anal intercourse. Differences appear in the way the recollections are expressed. Although the proportional indicators section in Table 6.5 presents the question in the format of a proportion, a proportion can also be calculated from questions 2 and 2b in the first section. In general, the advantages of such methods include ease of administration, economy, and ease of quantification and data analysis. The disadvantages lie in the recall ability of the participants, the reliability of responses, item clarity, the respondent's literacy level, and the degree to which items can be accurately translated from English into other languages.

Table 6.5. Three Indicators Used in Assessing
the Frequency of Insertive Anal Intercourse

Frequency counts[a]

1. Have you engaged in active anal intercourse in the past 2 months?

     _____ yes   _____ no

2. (If yes) How many times had you engaged in active anal intercourse?

     _____ number of times.

   How many of those times did you (enter number):

     _____ not use a rubber?

     _____ use a rubber?

Likert-type scale[a]

1. In the past two months have you engaged in insertive anal intercourse?

     _____ yes   _____ no

2. (If yes) How often did you use condoms during insertive anal intercourse (check the one answer that best describes your behavior)?

     _____ Every time

     _____ Usually

     _____ Sometimes

     _____ Seldom

     _____ Never

3. About how many times in the last 30 days did you have sex with your main male partner (check the one answer that best describes your behavior)?

     _____ Once in the last 30 days

     _____ Several times a day

     _____ Several times/last 30 days   _____ N/A

     _____ About once a week   _____ Not sure/DK

     _____ Several times a week   _____ Refused

     _____ Daily or almost daily

4. Of these times, how often did you have anal (insertive) sex (check the one answer that best describes your behavior)?

     _____ All of the time   _____ Never

     _____ Often   _____ N/A

     _____ Sometimes   _____ Not sure/DK

     _____ Rarely   _____ Refused

Proportional indicators[b]

1. Have you engaged in active anal intercourse in the past two months?

     _____ yes   _____ no

2. (If yes) What proportion of the time did you use a condom during active anal intercourse (check the one answer that best describes your behavior)?

     _____ None of the time

     _____ 25% of the time

     _____ 50% of the time

     _____ 75% of the time

     _____ 100% of the time

[a]From Mantell, Rapkin, Tross, & Ortíz-Torres (1992).
[b]From Martin (1985).

The relative merits of each approach are dependent on the data needs and the sophistication of the participants. Considering the proportion of time a respondent engages in a specific behavior allows the evaluator to measure the degree of consistency in behavior with different partners. Some people, however, have difficulty in grasping the concept of "proportion" outside of 100% or 0%. As such, trying to determine accurate percentages for behaviors that do not fall into either extreme often can lead to unreliable estimates of frequency. Outside of use with well-educated groups, proportional indicators can be problematic.

Likewise, frequency counts require detailed recall on the part of the participants. Requiring respondents to recall exact counts of many behaviors over a long period of time is particularly arduous.

STRATEGIES FOR IMPROVING MEASUREMENT OF ITEMS

The secret of a good scale lies in the clarity of the concept to be measured and the construction of items to measure it. With each potential item, the evaluator must ask what dimension of the construct of interest this item is tapping. An item or question is not a "snapshot" of the knowledge, attitudes, or behaviors under study. To take an efficient sample of items, each item should provide the evaluator with important and necessary information. Dead items (items that do not contribute to the total score) waste time. This section reviews the comprehensibility and language, specificity of measures, cultural sensitivity, clarity, retrospective assessment, equivalence of items across constructs, pretesting, and statistical means of addressing these issues.

Comprehensibility of Questionnaire Items

Constructing language-appropriate items for an evaluation requires knowledge of the target population. The wording of items must match the reading level of the target audience. It is insufficient to gear a questionnaire to a sixth-grade reading level (the usual suggested standard) if the population under study comes from a socioeconomic group who possesses a lower reading level than the population as a whole.

With certain populations, the use of pictures may be helpful. For example, a peer education program for Latinas that presented AIDS prevention information in the form of *pláticas* (talks or dialogues) used graphic illustrations to depict possible means of transmission and ways to protect themselves from AIDS (Arguelles, Rivero, Rhodes, & Wolitski, 1988). Several pictures from this questionnaire are presented in Fig. 6.2.

It is important to remember that much of the initial AIDS prevention work began in gay communities composed of primarily white, middle-class men. As a result, many of the terms frequently used with gay and bisexual men may be confusing or meaningless to other communities. For example, in GMHC's educational initiatives with residents in drug-free therapeutic communities, the phrase "negotiating for safer sex" was confusing—he notion that one "negotiates" for sex—to therapeutic community residents. Also, among low-income African-American women and Latinas, negotiating for safer sex may be

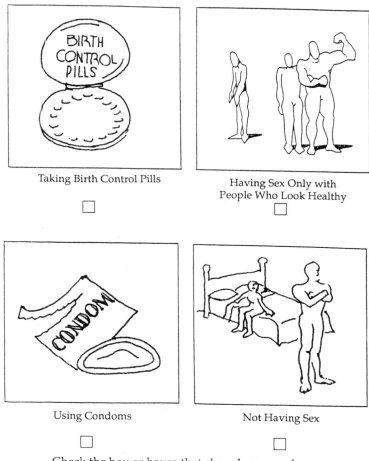

Taking Birth Control Pills

Having Sex Only with
People Who Look Healthy

Using Condoms

Not Having Sex

Check the box or boxes that show how people can
protect themselves from AIDS .

Figure 6.2. Graphic illustrations of modes of AIDS transmission and methods of protection. Adapted
from Arguelles, Rivero, Rhodes, & Wolitski, 1988, with permission.

nonexistent; many women do not have a choice and have sex in response to male
demands. Yet, this term has become a buzzword in HIV prevention programming.

Problems with terminology also occur with respect to measuring drug use. Persons
who purchase or rent previously used equipment, or "works," may view it as their
personal property, and hence are not "sharing" the needle per se. Further, persons who
share "works" with family or close friends also may not characterize themselves as
sharing equipment (Des Jarlais & Friedman, 1988). Wording questions in this manner
can lead to underestimation of needle sharing. Hence, it is important to keep in mind that
words and terms common to one group may not be readily comprehended by another.

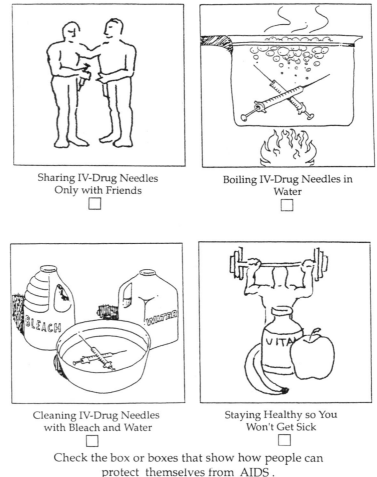

Sharing IV-Drug Needles
Only with Friends
☐

Boiling IV-Drug Needles in
Water
☐

Cleaning IV-Drug Needles
with Bleach and Water
☐

Staying Healthy so You
Won't Get Sick
☐

Check the box or boxes that show how people can
protect themselves from AIDS.

Figure 6.2. (*Continued*)

Specificity of Measures

Specificity of measures needs to be carefully considered in quantifying cognitive, attitudinal, and behavioral items. In general, items that are specific rather than global in nature are better predictors of outcomes. For example, if a researcher believes that assertiveness is a significant predictor of condom use, then the items should reflect sexual rather than general assertiveness, as shown in Example 6.7.

Also, questions about drug use and sexual behavior are better asked in terms of specific rather than summative behaviors, e.g., injection of specific drugs and vaginal intercourse with a condom versus injection of all drugs in a specific time period or

Retrospective Assessment

Sometimes, questionnaire items are written to assess participants' past behavior or attitudes. This is retrospective assessment. When determining the window period for assessment, respondents' recall capacity must be considered. For example, asking participants about their behaviors over the past week can yield fairly reliable responses, but provides limited information about stable or typical baseline information. If the questions involve a long period of time (the last 5 years or more or over lifetime), the reliability and validity of the responses are in serious question. For example, how many sexually active people actually know the exact number of times they have engaged in a given sexual act over the past 5 years? If drug users are asked to recall drug use over the last 5 to 10 years, it may be particularly difficult because many drugs affect users' memory. This may be further complicated by their use of multiple substances. Is it realistic to expect that drug users will remember how often and with whom they shared needles 7 years ago? Thus, this measure will not yield "clean" data.

It is generally a good idea to limit the window period for retrospection to between 2 weeks to 6 months (1 month is frequently used) to establish a meaningful baseline and help ensure reliable response patterns. This is referred to as time-bounding of measures. Using bold-faced type, italics, caps, or underlining to differentiate the time-bounded section from the rest of a question's text will draw a participant's or interviewer's attention to the window period. Example 6.9 presents a question with a 6-month referent.

Some data suggest that shorter recall periods for reporting of sexual activities provide the most consistent self-reported behavioral data (Kauth, St. Lawrence, & Kelly, 1991). While asking participants about their sexual behaviors over the past week should yield fairly reliable responses, information about typical practices is not provided. In general, the more specific the task required by the question (e.g., recalling frequency counts), the shorter the time period should be.

Some investigators have handled the problem of retrospective assessment in a unique way. Two interview survey studies (Martin, 1985; Becker & Joseph, 1988) conducted in the first decade of the epidemic required participants to recall their behaviors "the year before hearing about AIDS" ("pre-AIDS") and over the "past year." Participants were asked questions such as the one shown in Example 6.10. The question was later repeated to include the instructional set "over the past year."

As a means of guarding against response variation due to memory distortion, the researchers tried to "place the participant in the time period." Anchoring an item within

---

Example 6.9.   Time-Bounded Item

Overall, how satisfied have you been with your life for the *last six months*? Circle a number on the line below which best describes your level of satisfaction.

1	2	3	4	5	6
Very Dissatisfied					Very Satisfied

Example 6.10. Method of Determining Frequency of Behavior

Looking back to the year before you heard about AIDS, think of all the times you had sex during that year. How often did you use each drug when you had sex?

	Not used	1/4 time	1/2 time	3/4 time	Almost always
Marijuana, hashish (pot, grass)	1	2	3	4	5

(SOURCE: Martin, 1985.)

---

an historical context helps to provide a framework in which the participant can more accurately respond. Care must be taken, however, to ensure that the historical referent is not too long in the past. Other events and places, such as newsworthy stories and popular clubs, can also serve as memory triggers.

Finally, the Likert-type approach to assessment can be confusing if the intervals between the extremes are open to interpretation, as shown in question 2, second section, in Table 6.5. The difference between "sometimes" and "seldom" is subjective for each respondent. Given an equal probability of measurement error, measuring frequency of condom use with a Likert-type response yields a more imprecise estimate than do frequency counts. Using a focus group to pilot the instrument can be helpful in determining the clearest means by which to assess the frequency of behaviors.

Equivalence of Item Content across Constructs

Constructs refer to the underlying phenomenon or concept being measured. In the area of HIV prevention, a person's belief in his or her ability, or self-efficacy, to practice safer sex is an example of a construct. Likewise, a respondent's intent to perform a safer sex practice (behavior intention) is also a construct. The equivalence of the items (e.g., the identical wording of the root of the questions) across the concepts is a decision that the researcher must confront. If self-efficacy and behavioral intentions regarding condom use are going to be assessed, the items in these two scales should be equivalent, as shown in Example 6.11.

If an evaluator is interested in how well self-efficacy and condom intentions predict condom use following an intervention, then content equivalence is important. In statistical analysis (e.g., a regression equation), if self-efficacy is found to be a stronger predictor of condom use than intentions, one must be certain that this is not an artifact of differences in specific item content rather than due to the construct itself (Meyer-Bahlburg, 1995, personal communication). Otherwise, if assessment is geared toward informing intervention, different item content in the two constructs might be important.

Pretesting Instruments

Pretesting the proposed instruments with a small number of members of the target population in the field will provide immediate feedback about whether the issues

---

Example 6.11. Equivalence of Item Content across Constructs

Intentions:

In the coming 6 months, how likely is it that you will use a condom every time you have vaginal sex with your main partner?

Self-Efficacy:

How confident are you that you will use a condom every time for vaginal sex with your main partner?

Norms:

How many of the people you know use a condom every time they have vaginal sex with their main partner?

(SOURCE: U.S. Centers for Disease Control and Prevention, Division of STD/HIV, AIDS Community Demonstration Projects, HIV Prevention Interventions, 1991.)

---

described above are problematic. It is most effective when followed by discussion groups or individual interviews with participants to elicit specific feedback on how clear the items were and the degree to which the evaluator has met his or her goal in eliciting information through a particular item.

For example, GMHC research program staff pretested knowledge and assertiveness scales on a sample of therapeutic community residents, the purpose of which was to determine the language appropriateness of items, assess baseline knowledge for this community, and maximize scale utility. An item analysis indicated that certain areas of knowledge were universally understood by the participants, while the wording of some items was confusing or ambiguous to the respondents. This led to clarification of specific language issues and revision of the instrument.

Methodological Solutions to Improving Participant Response to Items

Multiple methodological and procedural options borrowed from large-scale social experiments can be applied to assessment of sexual behavior, drug use, and HIV status to elicit sensitive information (Boruch, 1988a). While these methods protect individuals' privacy and assure confidentiality, they have inherent methodological limitations and require field testing.

Some procedural options include conducting anonymous surveys, or using an intermediary to elicit information or to act as a broker, linking records by matching encoded information (except identifying information) from two independent sources (e.g., interview data with medical records) (Boruch & Cecil, 1979; Boruch, 1988a,b). With the latter strategy, however, evaluators need to be careful that an individual's identity cannot be deduced from the process used to match records.

In asking sensitive questions, another option would be to ask participants to use an alias. Tested individuals may be given the names of movie stars; each "movie star" would be assigned a week or month in which to return for notification of HIV test results, as done by the Seattle–King County Department of Health (R. Wood, personal communication).

SELECTING A SCALE OR INDEX: MAKING AN INFORMED CHOICE

Combining individual measurement points (items) can enable the evaluator to quantify an individual's knowledge, attitudes, and behaviors on subjects of interest. These areas include sexual activity, drug use, knowledge about HIV/AIDS, psychosocial issues such as fear of death and locus of control, and self-esteem. Armed with a battery of tests, the evaluator is able to determine the impact and outcome of a preventive health intervention.

In this section, we discuss what the evaluator should look for in the selection of an existing scale or index to ensure that he or she is assessing what was intended. Understanding item analysis, reliability and validity testing, and how an instrument is modified to meet the needs of a particular evaluation are the benchmarks for making an informed choice in selecting a quantitative instrument.

A *scale* refers to a collection of similar items that measure an area of interest that can be grouped and collapsed into a single meaningful composite score. Scales are often used to measure beliefs and attitudes, such as satisfaction with barrier methods or perceived vulnerability to HIV infection.

An *index* refers to the combining of several components of a construct and treating them as a single comprehensive measure. For example, 35 items measuring different aspects of AIDS-related knowledge (sexual transmission, maternal–infant transmission, drug-related transmission) represent a knowledge index.

The terms index and scale are often used interchangeably; however, they possess different psychometric properties. The index is an ordinal measure. By this, we mean that the evaluator is able to make comparisons among groups or individuals and assess change over time in terms of rank order differences. For example, if the intervention group correctly answered 50 items on a knowledge index and the comparison group answered 25 items correctly, an evaluator could say that as a function of program participation, the intervention group was significantly more knowledgeable about HIV transmission than the comparison group. However, the evaluator could not say that the intervention group was twice as knowledgeable as the comparison group.

A scale, which uses interval-like data, allows the evaluator to look at patterns of responses and to make interpretations that go beyond rank ordering. In utilizing a scale, the evaluator can make statements such as "the intervention group is twice as likely to use a condom than the comparison group." In general, scales are superior to indices, in that they permit more interpretation of the results. However, it is important to note that not everything that is labeled a scale is in fact a scale. For example, projects may refer to a knowledge test as a knowledge scale, when in fact it is an index.

Often it is better to use a scale or index developed by others than constructing new

Table 6.6. Items from an HIV/AIDS Knowledge Index
for Gay and Bisexual Men

Response	Item description
T F ?	1. Reducing the number of sex partners is the best way to lower your risk of AIDS.
T F ?	2. If you have been monogamous for 3 years, you do not need to practice safer sex.
T F ?	3. Rubbers, when used properly, can prevent the spread of the AIDS virus during cock sucking.
T F ?	4. HIV cannot get into the body through cuts in the skin.
T F ?	5. It is safe to suck cock as long as your partner does not cum in your mouth.
T F ?	6. A person already infected with HIV does not need to practice safer sex.
T F ?	7. The largest percentage of people with AIDS in the United States are gay and bisexual men.
T F ?	8. If drug users clean needles and works with bleach before sharing them, they reduce the risk of infecting each other with HIV.
T F ?	9. If a man is infected with HIV, there is no safe way to have sex with him.
T F ?	10. Condoms can be reused if washed thoroughly after use.
T F ?	11. Always blow up the condom with some air to check for any leaks or damage.

measures. This will save the evaluator time and resources as well as avoiding duplication of measures. Indices and scales are found in numerous places: the instrumentation section of empirical articles published in the public health and social science literature, measures identified through the evaluator's network with other researchers, and in special publications of instruments such as *Buros Mental Measurements Yearbook* and *Tests in Print* (Buros Institute for Mental Measurements, 1994, 1995).

Of utmost importance is the ability to evaluate the utility of the index or scale. Existing scales are often standardized on a population, with reliability and validity established. Other important considerations in selecting a preexisting scale are: (1) its frequency of use and on which populations; (2) whether it is appropriate for the target population; and (3) its ease of administration. We will look at two examples to illustrate these points.

Choosing an Index

Numerous indices have been used in the evaluation of interventions with various populations. In Table 6.6, there are 11 items from a 35-item knowledge index developed to assess the impact of an HIV prevention program for gay and bisexual men in New York City (Mantell *et al.*, 1989a). Each individual item is a simple measure of AIDS-related knowledge. Combined, the items provide a composite score, or index. The discussion of face validity, item variance, floor and ceiling effects, and reliability and validity applies to scales as well as indices.

Face Validity

The first question an evaluator would ask is, "Does this index apply to the group I'm working with?" In other words, are the items in the index culturally competent for the group in question. A related issue is whether the wording of the items appear related to knowledge about HIV/AIDS. This is referred to as face validity, and it addresses whether or not the instrument appears to measure what it is intended to measure. A test of AIDS-related knowledge should have questions about transmission modes, prevalence, prevention, drug use, and sexual behaviors.

Face validity is an important first step in determining the suitability of a measure. If the scales do not appear valid, it may be difficult to secure participants' compliance. This is particularly important in trying to adapt a scale designed for one population for use with another. For example, if you have an AIDS-related knowledge scale developed for adolescents and want to use it for adults, its language and examples could insult the audience, who might refuse to finish the test or not take it seriously. Having a test appear valid is a necessary, yet insufficient, means of establishing face validity.

Item Variance

Another point of consideration is how well the knowledge index differentiates among a group being tested. This is determined by the item variance (i.e., the varying response patterns of respondents across an item). The purpose of an index in evaluation is to differentiate among participants, for example, who benefited from the program and who did not. As a result, not everyone should score the same on the test. In the absence of variation among participants, statistical testing of data becomes meaningless. For example, in an AIDS knowledge test the items should reflect real differences in the knowledge base of the population under study. In a true–false test, the greatest discrimination occurs when 50% of the sample answers true and 50% answers false.

The variance in a dichotomous item is found by multiplying the proportion correct by the proportion incorrect. The 50–50 split results in the greatest value, as shown in Table 6.7. Varied degrees of difficulty provide for a variance in scores and make a test challenging (though not too frustrating) for the participant.

Floor and Ceiling Effects

The consideration of item variance is directly related to avoiding the pitfall of floor and ceiling effects. Instruments that produce skewed results where everyone scores at the bottom of the index (floor effect) or the top of the index (ceiling effect) become unusable in an evaluation. Floor effects occur for multiple reasons. First, in a knowledge test with too many difficult items, all respondents will end up with a low score. In this instance, the test fails to discriminate among respondents. Likewise, knowledge scales with items that are too easy will yield the same lack of variability; however, this time the scores will be at the high end, or ceiling, of the scale. It is important to note that a ceiling effect may be an index construction problem or it may reflect a reality of the community being assessed— that the community's knowledge is so high that everyone will be at the ceiling of the index.

Reliability

In evaluating the utility of an index, the evaluator must assess the index's reliability. The reliability of a measure refers to the consistency of its scores over time. An observed

Table 6.7. Possible Values
of Item Variance

Proportion correct	Proportion incorrect	Item variance
.5	.5	.25
.4	.6	.24
.3	.7	.21
.2	.8	.16
.1	.9	.09

test score (X) is composed of a person's true score (T) and measurement error (E). Measurement error is anything contributing to a person's score that does not reflect that which was intended. The reliability of a test is an index of the true test score. For example, if you had a watch that on the average lost 2 minutes every hour, this instrument would be unreliable as a measurer of time.

There are four basic ways to assess the reliability of a measure. These are (1) inter-rater, (2) internal consistency, (3) test–retest, and (4) alternate forms reliability. Table 6.8

Table 6.8. Types of Reliability

Type of reliability	Description
Interrater	• Provides an estimate of the agreement between at least two trained independent judges who rate the same individual's test results or narrative comments using the same criteria. Resulting coefficient reflects objectivity of scoring. • Often used in quantification of qualitative data. • Issues of temporal fluctuations or content sampling are not addressed.
Internal consistency	• Assesses the degree to which items are related to each other and to the total score itself. Correlation between components of the test reflects the internal consistency of responses (e.g., Spearman-Brown Kuder-Richardson formula 20, and Cronbach's alpha). • Assumes that: (1) the items are homogeneous (all sample the same domain); (2) the scale score is unidimensional (only one construct is being measured); and (3) the data are either dichotomous (a 0/1 forced-choice format) or follow an interval-type scale (e.g., Likert-type).
Test–retest	• Assesses the relative agreement between two administrations of the same test to the same group of individuals at two points in time. • Indicates instrument's stability over time, i.e., how much test scores can be generalized over different occasions. • Testing intervals should be between a few weeks to a maximum of 6 months.
Alternate forms	• Create an equivalent form of the test, using different items, and has the same people fill out both forms. • Assesses the degree to which two sets of scores agree. • Indicates both temporal stability and consistency of instrument across different item samples. • Reduces variation in participant's score due to rehearsal or practice effects.

outlines these four forms. For knowledge indices, internal consistency reliability is the method of choice. If you developed a test aimed at measuring one construct or knowledge area, you would expect that, on the average, a person will perform the same way on each item of the test. In other words, the items should all be highly related to each other and to the total score itself. Internal consistency reliability is the measure of this interrelationship.

Internal consistency reliability is predicated on the following assumptions: the items are homogeneous (all sample the same domain), the scale score is unidimensional (only one construct is being measured), and the data are either dichotomous (a 0–1 forced-choice format) or follow an interval-type scale, such as a Likert-type scale. The test is analyzed such that the subdivisions of items are treated as alternate forms of the same test. Correlation between components of the test reflects the internal consistency, or the reliability, of responses.

There are many formulas and procedures available to obtain estimates of the internal consistency. The Spearman–Brown formula and Kuder–Richardson formula 20 are two examples. The most commonly used method, however, is to calculate Cronbach's alpha. This method creates a statistical equivalent of a parallel form for a test. A correlation coefficient is calculated, comparing the test with its "statistical clone." High values for alpha indicate high internal consistency. Near-zero values indicate low internal consistency. Low alpha values can mean either that the test is unreliable or that it is tapping more than one dimension. It is often necessary to apply other techniques to determine if the test is actually measuring more than one construct.

An important benefit of Cronbach's alpha is that it will provide the correlation between each item and the total test score. You can then determine which items contribute to the test score and which diminish the reliability of the scale. Based on an a priori decision, items with low correlation to the total test score (e.g., < 0.35, or < 0.50) would be dropped and the analysis rerun. Table 6.9 shows the interitem correlations for the 11 items from the knowledge index.

Based on the 35 items in the original measure, the index was shown to be highly reliable (alpha $= 0.9875$). It was also shown that two of the items correlated poorly with the others. Item 1, "Reducing the number of sex partners is the best way to lower your risk of AIDS" and item 11, "Always blow up the condom with some air to check for any leaks or damage," had an interitem correlation of 0.5199 and 0.5203, respectively. In each case, the alpha coefficient would have been slightly higher without the item.

However, the reliability of a scale is based on the number of items and their configuration at the time of testing. A test is altered by dropping items; in effect, creating a new scale. As there is no way to determine what impact these two items had on participants' response patterns, the new scale, excluding the two items, needs to be subjected to the same reliability analysis as the original scale.

Test–retest reliability can be established by administering an instrument at 1- to 4-week intervals to a small sample. Choosing a small sample for readministration will help keep the costs down. Interrater reliability of an instrument can be established by having a panel of at least two expert judges assess an instrument. Reliability is obtained by determining the level of agreement among the raters. This is discussed in greater detail in Chapter 7 on qualitative assessment.

is a data-reduction technique, i.e., a means of reducing a large number of questionnaire items to a fewer number based on the researcher's interpretation of the meaning of the construct. For example, with this technique, a set of 25 items can be grouped and condensed into three factors, which are then used to create scales. Ideally, an item will load or belong on one factor and not load highly on any other (DeVellis, 1991). A factor loading is a value between −1.0 and +1.0 and is interpreted similar to a correlation coefficient as the measure of the relationship between the items and the factor. A loading of at least .4 is often used as a cutoff point to determine whether an item loads on a particular factor.

The pattern by which items load on factors is called the *factor structure*. If an item loads .8671 on factor 1 and .1062 on factor 2, this item belongs with factor 1 rather than factor 2. The use of varimax factor rotation will reduce the likelihood of items loading on more than one factor and will result in independent factors. The evaluator can allow the computer to choose the number of factors or he or she can choose a priori based on some theoretical rationale.

Different factors measure different constructs in a set of items. By examining the items that make up different factors, a researcher is able to label each factor. Validity for the different scales that emerge is a combination of statistical technique and the judgment of the evaluator.

The 17-item modified Rand Social Support Scale was administered to 306 gay men, and a factor analysis was performed on the data. The resultant structure indicated three factors (see Table 6.13). The first factor was comprised of eight items, whose item content

Table 6.13. Representation of the Factor Structure of the Social Support Scale[a,b]

Item	Factor 1	Factor 2	Factor 3
Someone (SO) to listen to you	*****		
SO to confide in	*****		
SO to tell worries	*****		
SO who understands	*****		
SO who gives good advice	*****		
SO who gives information	*****		
SO whose advice you want	*****		
SO to turn to for suggestions	*****		
SO who shows love and affection		*****	
SO who hugs you		*****	
SO to love/make feel wanted		*****	
SO who can lend you money			*****
SO to cook your meals			*****
SO to do your laundry			*****
SO to move in with			*****
So to call in case of emergencies			*****
SO to shop for you			*****

[a]From Mantell *et al.* (1989b).
[b]*****, Represents significant factor loading.

represented availability of resources or information. The second factor included three items, their content indicating availability of emotional support. Finally, the six-item third factor addressed the availability of tangible support. The strength and clarity of the factor structure lent support to the construct validity of this scale. Hence, the two original scales were retained and the hypothesized third scale was demonstrated as valid.

As with any measurement instrument, modification requires the evaluator to reestablish the reliability of the instrument. Since the social support scale in question is actually three subscales, reliability for each subscale was calculated. A Cronbach's alpha was determined for each subscale, indicating reliability scores in the 0.90s. This indicated that the subscales were reliable as well as valid.

MEASUREMENT ERROR

The degree to which items do not measure what the evaluator intends can be called measurement error. The impact of measurement error is far reaching, in that it can lead to findings that are both confusing and misleading and ultimately open to misinterpretation. The reduction of measurement error in an index or scale increases the instruments reliability and its validity. Reduction of measurement error also clarifies the interpretableness of results, leading to a cleaner assessment of the variables under study.

Assessment of sexual behaviors (e.g., the number of partners; frequency of anal, oral, and vaginal intercourse with and without condoms; masturbation; and the use of sex toys) is problematic in AIDS research (Catania, Gibson, Marin, Coates, & Greenblatt, 1990a; Catania *et al.*, 1993). The researcher generally is unable to observe sexual interactions, and therefore cannot verify that the behavior actually took place. Using the incidence of STDs as an indicator of sexual activity will underestimate the frequency of unprotected sex because individuals may be unaware that they have an STD, or even if they suspect or are aware, may not seek definitive diagnosis and treatment. Some researchers have implemented condom redemption programs in which participants are given coupons to exchange for condoms as an indicator of intentions to engage in protected sex (Rickert, Gottlieb, & Jay, 1990). This method is limited in that it neither reflects actual use nor indicates the type of sexual activity for which condoms will be used.

Some potential sources of measurement bias are nonresponse, difficulty recalling events, sociodemographic characteristics, emotional state and extent of perceived threat in relation to that behavior, data collection method, how the questions are asked, order of questions and question context, and an interviewer's sociodemographic characteristics and comfort level in asking questions, particularly about sex. As noted by Catania and colleagues (1993), measurement error can lead to: (1) unreliable estimates of the prevalence of high-risk sexual behaviors in a population; (2) misidentification of at-risk populations; and (3) biased estimates of interrelationships among variables. Table 6.14 identifies some of the causes of measurement error in the assessment of sexual and drug-related behaviors. For a more detailed discussion of measurement error, see Catania *et al.* (1993).

Whether the evaluator is creating a new measure, modifying an existing measure, or using an existing measure in its entirety, he or she must establish the measure's utility for the population under study. This requires some psychometric analysis of the measure. The case study below describes a psychometric study of a scale to measure the safer sex practices of adolescents and young adults. Sources of measurement error are identified and controlled to increase the soundness of the instrument. Special attention is paid to item construction and the determination of the instrument's reliability and validity.

CASE STUDY OF PSYCHOMETRIC ANALYSES OF A SAFER SEX SCALE

DiIorio, Parsons, Lehr, Adame, and Carlone (1992) constructed the Safe Sex Behavior Questionnaire (SSBQ) for use with college freshmen. The investigators began by identifying the dimensions of safer sex through a content analysis of the pamphlet *Understanding AIDS*, which was sent to all households in the United States by the Surgeon General's Office, US Department of Health and Human Services, in 1988. Four domains were identified: (1) barrier protection during intercourse; (2) avoidance of high

Table 6.14. Sources of Measurement Error Related to Assessing the Effectiveness of HIV/AIDS Prevention Programs

Source of error	Reduction of error
Sensitivity of questions	The sensitive nature of questions regarding sex and substance use practices may lead to participants responding in socially desirable ways. Questions must be posed such that respondents are able to answer honestly.
Defining the terminology	Error occurs when the evaluator assumes everyone defines terms in the same way. It is necessary to define what is being asked (e.g., rather than referring to safer sex, refer to specific rather than global risk-reduction behaviors).
Assumptions about target population	Construction of items based on preconceived ideas about the behaviors and motivations of the target population can lead to results that are biased and misleading. Items should allow for broad-based responses including responses not "typically" associated with the population (e.g., heterosexuals engaging in same-sex behavior).
Assessing partner type	With whom the behavior is engaged is as important as assessing what behaviors the respondent engages in. It has been found that condom use varies if the partner is a steady vs. casual one. Failure to examine the effects of partner status can mask important differences in relationships between variables.
Response format	The choice of response categories, or metric of questions, affects the measurement precision. Having too many or too few response categories can become confusing for the respondent. For example, the choice of *safe*, *possibly safe*, or *unsafe* may obscure important differences, because three choices are insufficient to indicate the true spread of responses.
Retrospective assessment	Time-bounding retrospective assessments provides the respondent with a frame of reference for more accurate responding.
Cultural sensitivity and competence	Language of items must accommodate the cultural values and norms of the populations being surveyed.
Specificity of items	Each item should measure only one thing. Ambiguous or "double-barreled" items result in unusable data (e.g., Do you believe you can shoot drugs without sharing needles? is ambiguous in that *no* can mean either you have to share needles or you do not engage in shooting drugs).

risk behaviors; (3) avoidance of bodily fluids; and (4) interpersonal skills (e.g., negotiation and assertiveness). From these domains a pool of 35 items was constructed. Using a roundtable discussion approach, the pool was reduced to 27 items. Seventeen items were worded in the positive direction and ten were in the negative. Each item was rated on a four-point, Likert-type scale ranging from 1 = never to 4 = always. Total scores range from 27 to 108 in the direction of safer sex practices.

Content validity was established using three experts in the field of public health. Each item was reviewed for meaning, clarity, and unidimensionality. In addition, each item was rated on its relationship to safer sex. A validity index of 98% was obtained, indicating a high degree of agreement among the raters. A sample of 89 sexually active freshman was identified in a nonrandom convenience sample of registrants in a freshman seminar class. Cronbach's alpha indicated an internal consistency rating of .82.

Factor analysis on two independent samples of men and women indicated similar five-structure solutions. Among men, the five factors were: (1) use of condoms, (2) homosexual practices, (3) use of assertiveness skills, (4) avoidance of bodily fluids, and (5) avoidance of risky behaviors. For women, the factor structure included: (1) avoidance of anal intercourse, (2) use of condoms, (3) use of assertiveness skills, (4) avoidance of risky behaviors, and (5) avoidance of bodily fluids. For the men, internal consistency measures ranged from 0.52 to 0.84 with alpha = 0.80 for the total scale score, and for women the range was 0.52 to 0.84 (alpha = 0.83 for total scale score). On independent samples of men and women, test–retest reliability was performed. Similar findings were found for men and women.

Construct validation of the scale was performed on another sample. It was hypothesized that the construct safe sex behavior would be negatively correlated with the construct risk-taking behavior (high risk-takers would score low on dimensions of safe sex) and positively correlated with the construct assertiveness (assertive people would be more likely to practice safe sex). Participants were asked to complete the SSBQ, the College Self-Expression Scale (CSES), a measure of general assertiveness, and the Risk-Taking Questionnaire (RTQ). The general hypotheses were supported among both the male and female sample. Among men, the SSBQ was significantly correlated with both the CSES and the RTQ (0.39 and −0.34, respectively). Among women, significant correlations in the predicted directions were also found (0.27 and −0.21, respectively).

The authors pointed out the need for further testing of the instrument with more heterogeneous samples to determine if the factor structures can be replicated and whether the relatively low reliability indexes could be increased (DiIorio et al., 1992).

Although this type of rigor in scale construction is rarely applied in the evaluation of HIV/AIDS preventive interventions, it is vital for their evaluation. Without repeated testing and refinement of questionnaires and scales, the validity of evaluation findings comes under serious question.

CONCLUSION

Instruments for quantitative evaluation of HIV/AIDS preventive interventions are only as good as the items that make them up. There are many means of trying to tap an

3. Construction–enumeration. Qualitative research entails a process of abstraction in which units of analysis become apparent and are discovered over the course of observation. Data are often not reduced into numeric form. In contrast, quantitative methods focus on counting predetermined or observed variables or units of analysis.
4. Subjectivity–objectivity. In qualitative research, the focus is on the perspective of the people under study. Categories derived from participants' experiences are reconstructed. In quantitative research, researchers rely on conceptual categories developed by external observers to analyze unique populations.

Bogdan and Biklen (1982) identify two other characteristics frequently associated with the use of qualitative research paradigms: (1) occurrence in natural settings; and (2) an orientation toward process as well as outcomes. Both of these attributes, however, may also be features of quantitative paradigms.

The distinction between qualitative and quantitative methods is not always clear-cut. Some data collection strategies, such as diaries, vignettes/scenarios, medical/social service records, and surveys, can be both qualitative and/or quantitative. Whether they are qualitative or quantitative, will depend on whether their response categories are open- or closed-ended. In this chapter, discussion is limited to their qualitative application. (The quantitative application of these methods has been addressed in Chapter 6.)

Qualitative assessment in evaluation research can include the use of open-ended questions in structured surveys, unstructured interviews, in-depth direct observation, and group methods such as focus groups, the nominal group process, and the Delphi method (a method that has both qualitative and quantitative features). The latter two are consensus-building techniques that entail ranking participants' opinions. Vignettes/scenarios, diaries, ethnographic approaches, and medical/social service record reviews are other commonly used qualitative strategies. The actual applications of these diverse qualitative methods vary greatly due to the expertise of research personnel, number of participants, time line, costs, and settings, as well as desired results.

RATIONALE FOR USING QUALITATIVE METHODS

Qualitative research is particularly appropriate for answering questions related to processes of program implementation, how and why a program works, as well as for understanding unintended outcomes and participants' behaviors. It can provide an in-depth understanding of the nature of personal experiences about which little is known, a new perspective on events about which a great deal is known, as well as illustrate or clarify quantitative study findings.

Qualitative evaluation techniques are especially effective for eliciting information about sensitive AIDS-related issues (e.g., sexual practices and partnerships, drug use, stigma) not captured adequately with closed-ended questionnaire items. Opportunities for probing, asking follow-up questions, and interaction between the researcher and participants are afforded. Authenticity of participant voice is emphasized. Greater emphasis is placed on describing the reasons why program participants hold certain convictions or behave in a particular manner than on characterizing the numbers who share certain beliefs, behaviors, or sets of characteristics. For example, while it is necessary to know how often participants consistently use condoms during sexual intercourse, such information is insufficient to develop responsive HIV/AIDS preventive interventions.

With qualitative evaluation methods, the details of what happens within a particular preventive intervention, activity, or community are exposed. Discerning context is central to understanding participants' experiences. The researcher can delve deeper and therefore develop greater insight of participants' opinions, attitudes, values, and behaviors within specific contexts, e.g., under what circumstances people are able or unable to use condoms; how beliefs about HIV/AIDS and actual condom use vary between women in the informal sector (e.g., selling flowers or fruit) and those who are civil servants; how couples decide to contracept, choose a method, or have another child; how familial and partner support for HIV prevention influences women's HIV precautionary behavior; or why sexually active adolescents who do not use condoms believe they are invulnerable to HIV infection.

With quantitative survey methods, an evaluator can determine how many people use a specific HIV/AIDS service and present the data numerically (e.g., 45% of the 50 clients interviewed identified lack of transportation as a barrier to clinic attendance, or 95% of the sample watched the public service announcement on television regarding how to prevent HIV with the use of female barrier methods). In contrast, using a qualitative approach, an evaluator might convene a small group of people who normally use an HIV clinic and facilitate discussion on the meaning of HIV in their lives and their perceptions of the barriers to service delivery and care. The evaluator would then analyze these data by looking for recurring themes and supplementing them with specific quotations from participants. Developing explanations of these barriers is emphasized.

In the absence of preexisting standardized questionnaires with established reliability and validity, qualitative methods can be utilized to generate items for the development of quantitative instruments. For example, as discussed later in this chapter, focus groups are commonly conducted to create structured measures. They are also useful in generating a range of perspectives or viewpoints on specific issues from participants.

VALIDITY ISSUES IN QUALITATIVE DATA

There has often been an uneasiness about qualitative studies because they are seen as exploratory, subjective, and lacking scientific rigor (Denzin & Lincoln, 1994). Because events, e.g., observing a conversation between two people or reading open-ended responses from interviews or diaries, are interpreted by the researcher, their objectivity and internal validity or credibility have been questioned. The degree to which findings from a qualitative study can be extrapolated to larger populations, i.e., their external validity or transferability, depends in part on the characteristics of the sample and settings and how members were recruited and the precision of problem formulation and questions posed. For example, program evaluation based on one case within a setting lacks generalizability. However, since qualitative research often aims to be generative rather than verificative, generalizability to other groups (i.e, external validity) is not always a desired goal. Applying data from one specific context to another may actually invalidate the data.

Having reliable and internally valid data that are not idiosyncratic strengthen the credibility of the research (Goetz & LeCompte, 1984). Verifying conclusions about the data are as important as making the conclusions. This might require the researcher to look back at the data, confirm findings with another population, or attempt to achieve consensus by discussing findings with colleagues not involved in the research (Miles & Huberman, 1994). A series of techniques can be employed to enhance internal validity of qualitative study findings. Methods to improve accuracy and integrity of findings include: (1) cross-checking interpretation of findings by using other sources of data and methods, i.e., triangulation (Denzin, 1989), for example, comparing the results of in-depth interviews with those of a quantitative survey; (2) using multiple observers or raters to confirm or achieve consensus regarding study themes and findings (i.e., interrater or interobserver reliability); (3) repeated observations over varying conditions (e.g., by time, place, and gender of researchers) to determine if findings are consistent (Adler & Adler, 1994); (4) use of peer debriefers (Lincoln & Guba, 1985); (5) auditing, i.e., an external review of the analyses to document sources of bias in the data (Huberman & Miles, 1994); (6) obtaining feedback from participants; and (7) using tape or video recorders (Goetz & LeCompte, 1984).

APPLICATION OF QUALITATIVE METHODS

In this section, the features as well as advantages and disadvantages of various qualitative methods that can be applied to evaluation of HIV/AIDS programs are described. Examples are provided. These methods include: (1) open-ended questions on surveys; (2) in-depth unstructured interviews; (3) medical/social service records; (4) self-report diaries; (5) vignettes; (6) observational measures; (7) ethnography; (8) the nominal group process; (9) the Delphi technique; and (10) focus groups.

Open-Ended Questions on Surveys

Open-ended questions on surveys are the simplest type of qualitative assessment, consisting of questions that cannot be answered with a "yes" or "no" or from a menu of preselected responses. The respondent, with no cues or prompts provided by the researcher, answers the question based on whatever response occurs to him or her at the time. Respondents express answers in "their own words." This format allows respondents to describe their feelings, beliefs, attitudes, and behaviors without being confined or led by a structured question with limited response choices. Table 7.1 provides several illustrations of open-ended questions that can be used to elicit information about HIV/AIDS preventive beliefs and behaviors.

When included in predominantly quantitative surveys, open-ended items enhance

Table 7.1.   Examples of Open-Ended Questions

- Under what circumstances do you use and not use condoms?
- Why do you believe you are at high risk for HIV infection?
- How do you choose a sexual partner?
- What do you do to clean your needles?
- What were your main reasons for getting (not getting) tested for HIV?

an evaluation in two ways. First, by allowing participants a forum in which to express themselves, the evaluator is better able to make the numbers from quantitative results more meaningful. Asking participants when they would not use a condom can provide important information about motivational, partner-related, and situational determinants of nonuse. Elucidation of these factors will help focus data collection about frequency of condom use and suggest additional questions to be asked. Second, open-ended questions can make the data collection process more responsive and enjoyable for participants; their opinions will be recorded as they present them.

Disadvantages of Method

There are drawbacks, nonetheless, to asking open-ended questions. Typically, at the analysis stage, the raw qualitative responses are judged and categorized by skilled research staff to fall into one or more designated categories. At least two judges are needed. Since research analysts' biases can determine how categories are established, their development and how responses are assigned to them are assessed for interrater reliability, i.e., a consensus among at least two judges. This will improve the objectivity of the coding scheme. Interrater reliability among the judges can be assessed through the independent development of categories based upon agreed standards or response attributes early on in the data review process, such as at pretest. This will reduce the bias in the process by which responses are assigned to any particular response category.

Another way to lessen bias would be to include a broad spectrum of categories. An array of categories provides coders with greater direction for classification. For example, in classifying sexual risk behavior, three categories—high, moderate, and low risk—are subjected to the coders' interpretation. If there is controversy among AIDS providers as to the degree of risk of specific sexual behaviors, coders may have to rely more heavily on their own judgment of risk. However, if the researcher specifies ten codes reflecting different types of sexual intercourse (e.g., unprotected vaginal intercourse, unprotected insertive anal intercourse, unprotected receptive anal intercourse, unprotected insertive oral intercourse, unprotected receptive oral intercourse, protected vaginal intercourse, protected insertive anal intercourse, protected receptive anal intercourse, protected insertive oral intercourse, protected receptive oral intercourse) and attaches the degree of risk associated with each of these acts, the coders can be guided to more consistent classification. It is easier to collapse many categories into fewer ones after the data are coded than it is to expand or recapture data thereafter.

The possibility of bias is present in every analysis. Establishment of a reliable and standard method of codifying data can help alleviate this problem. Once the coding strategy has been established, training of coders is necessary to ensure everyone is coding in the same manner. Further, review by a designated researcher is essential to ensure that data are being coded consistently by the different raters, i.e., interrater reliability. Checking open-ended responses for consistency of interpretation in a random number of questionnaires while coding will improve quality control of the data. An in-depth explanation of techniques to reduce and report the data are discussed later in this chapter in the section on qualitative data analysis.

In-Depth Unstructured Interviews

Unlike structured or semistructured questions in surveys, in-depth unstructured interviews are open-ended and flexible and use follow-up questions (or probes) to elicit greater detail and explanations. Characterized by Kahn and Cannell (1957) as "conversations with a purpose," they follow a general set of goals, but include no structured questions and response categories.

The extent to which the questions are unstructured, however, can vary. An interview guide, which elaborates a list of topics, is used to frame the interview. This format provides participants with greater freedom to respond as if they were talking with the interviewer, presenting ideas in a style and in words with which they are comfortable (Marshall & Rossman, 1989). The interviewer can respond to unanticipated topics as they emerge during the course of the interview. Thus, in-depth unstructured interviews provide a forum for interactive participation of the interviewer and the person being interviewed, allowing for maximum exploration of a participant's attitudes and values. Interviews are conducted by personnel trained in the interactive process.

Interviews may be single or multiple, depending on the research objective (Conrad, 1990). With multiple or serial interviews, the processes associated with maintenance and relapse of sexual and drug-use risk-reduction behaviors can be monitored over time. Such information can be used to develop appropriately staged interventions based on participants' readiness to adopt precautionary behaviors. Also, the illness trajectory of a person with HIV infection, particularly the changing physical and psychological status and social and economic circumstances, can be captured.

Data collected from these interviews serve a variety of purposes, including: (1) characterizing HIV-related health beliefs, motivations, and behavioral processes; (2) generating survey questions and research hypotheses (Williams *et al.*, 1990); (3) suggesting the structure and content of interventions; and (4) evaluating programs and planning future programs. For example, through identification of themes, patterns, and trends, information about individuals' or a community's health-related beliefs, values, norms, behaviors, and hidden codes of conduct is collected to help design culturally sensitive HIV prevention programs (Newman, 1987). Among Latinas, areas for inquiry might include level of acculturation, patterns of sexual partnerships, social meanings attached to gender and sexuality, attitudes about pregnancy, contraception, injecting practices and rituals associated with sharing needles, and the structure and mobilization of support systems. Among rural women in South Africa, in-depth interviews will be helpful in understanding the symbolic language they use to refer to sexual organs and sexual intercourse, types of sexual partnerships (monogamous or casual), sexual risk behaviors, perceptions of the male condom and resistance to their use, and how to introduce the female condom into their communities.

Case Example: Reproductive Beliefs and Motivations. The New York City Department of Health's Perinatal HIV Prevention Project (Mantell, Ramos, DiVittis, & Whittier, 1989d)

With the risk of maternal–infant HIV transmission (about 15–25% of all babies born to HIV-infected women in the United States not treated with zidovudine are infected with HIV), interest in reproductive-related issues surrounding these women has heightened. Providers frequently assume that women will not choose to bear children if they are infected. They may find it difficult to fathom why pregnant women, knowing that they are infected and the risk of perinatal transmission, would continue their pregnancy. Many providers would consider such behavior to be socially irresponsible.

In-depth unstructured interviews with HIV-infected individuals or those at high risk for HIV can be used profitably to understand reproductive attitudes and behaviors with regard to HIV-infected women and men. Male and female drug users in methadone maintenance treatment were interviewed to explore meanings, behavior patterns, and processes underlying reproductive and contraceptive decision-making and the social and cultural contexts in which they occur. The interview guide for men focused on general life history, contraception and its relationship to fatherhood, the impact of pregnancy on the relationship, fatherhood, HIV testing, and partner contact notification. Questions relating to the topic of fatherhood in the male interview guide are presented in Table 7.2.

Data from these interviews served to modify the content of the preventive intervention for this population. For example, the finding that the men lacked knowledge about how specific contraceptive methods prevented pregnancy led to the incorporation of this topic in the intervention curricula.

Example 7.1 demonstrates the use of unstructured interview data for the Baltimore City Health Department's Community Dialogue Program (CDP) (Bentley & Santelli, 1990). The objective of the CDP was to ascertain why and how young people make decisions about using contraception and avoiding pregnancy and to identify specific health education strategies and messages to encourage responsible sexual decision-making.

Table 7.2. Interview Guide regarding Fatherhood Issues for Men[a]

Fatherhood
- What do men like/dislike about being a father?
- How important is it for a man to have children?
- If a man is not living with his partner, do they still have rights/duties as a father? What are they? How are they negotiated/maintained? If a child is not supported financially, does a man "give up" his paternity?
- What would you tell a man who wants to have a child?
- If you have a choice about the next baby you have, what would you like it to be? Boy or girl? Why?

[a]From Mantell, Kenny, & Cortez (1989c).

Example 7.1. Use of Unstructured Interviews for Program Planning:
The Community Dialogue Project, Baltimore City Department of Health

---

Unstructured interviews were conducted to garner information about teens' knowledge, attitudes, motivations, and behaviors concerning sexuality and contraception, relationship and dating patterns, and parenting. A convenience sample of 114 male and female teenagers yielded 91 interviews between April and July 1990.

Study findings indicated that the pill and the condom were the most frequent methods used by teens. Fear of AIDS was prevalent. Few teens reported regular condom use, and among those who used condoms, preventing AIDS was often a major incentive. As one 19-year-old male said: "I hear of this disease called AIDS and I am afraid of it ... so I use it [a condom] because I'm afraid of it."

Peer pressure was a major motivational determinant for engaging in sexual intercourse. According to one female teen, "You don't have your friends actually yelling at you to have sex ... but if you know your friends are sexually active and you want to be, even if they aren't forcing you to have sex, you just want to be one of them, so you have sex."

Having sex was spontaneous and unplanned, and consequently was a barrier to contraceptive use: "It wasn't something that was talked about. One minute you're sitting here talking and the next minute you're having sex. It just gradually happened, like I said, and I was just going with the flow."

(SOURCE: Bentley & Santelli, 1990.)

These interview data yielded important information for the design of pregnancy-planning campaigns targeted to adolescents. Based on these interview data, three recommendations for developing messages for adolescent pregnancy-planning campaigns were made: (1) provide an incentive for teens to use condoms regularly; (2) promote the value of condoms in preventing AIDS as well as teen pregnancy so as to increase condom use; and (3) ensure that teens have access to support networks to help them deal with sexuality and contraception.

Disadvantages of Method

Despite the benefits of unstructured interviews, the trade-offs of using this method must be considered. Due to the potential length and variety of responses, this technique relies heavily on an interviewer's skills and experiences to obtain usable data. Unless interviewers are well trained, the use of probes may appear to be unnecessary nuisance questions and potentially result in a negative subject–researcher interaction. Interviewers who lack knowledge of the participants' culture, are unfamiliar with the topic, are uncomfortable probing for information, or are poor listeners will have difficulty in obtaining usable data. Also, interviewers must be skilled in capturing the data, either on tape or by taking thorough notes. Role-playing and conducting a mock interview can help to assure an interviewer's level of familiarity with the research instruments and anticipate participants' behavior.

In-depth unstructured interviews are not only expensive to develop, implement, and analyze, but require considerable amounts of highly skilled staff time and effort. Transcribing a 1-hour audiotaped interview may require 3 to 4 hours, and analyzing responses to open-ended questions will demand months. In-depth interviews must be developed and administered with thought about how the data will be used. Finally, when conducted with a small number of respondents, they should not be used to make broad generalizations.

Medical/Social Service Records

Data collected from preexisting records from institutions and health care facilities, as noted previously, can provide the evaluator with both qualitative and quantitative data. When a clinical record review focuses on collecting frequency data, such as the number of different symptoms, the number of STD episodes, and medication regimens, as part of a detailed health history, they are quantitative in nature. However, when a nurse documents his or her subjective perceptions of a patient's agitation, they are qualitative. Once the data are coded, they are usually easy to analyze. Qualitative record data can also be used to cross-check information provided by participants in other research formats, such as comparing a nurse's subjective assessments of patients' psychological state with patients self-reports on a quantitative depression scale.

When program participants reside in institutions, e.g., prisons or drug-free therapeutic communities, a qualitative chart review can generate measures for impact evaluation. Notes from drug counselors and case managers can provide data about participants' affective states, social ties and interactions with therapeutic community peers, perceived adequacy of social support, and sexual risk behavior.

Disadvantages of Method

There are several problems associated with data collection from institutional records. First, such records are confidential and often require additional release forms signed by both the participant and an authorized representative of the institution. When sensitive information, such as HIV status, is in the records, patient consent may be low. Even when obtained, record data will only be as good as the recorder's skills. Often, the information is subjective (a counselor "feels" a client has an "attitude problem"), incomplete, and retrospective. Training staff on consistent and uniform methods of recording will improve completeness of documentation. In addition, this should improve interrater reliability, and hence, the internal validity of the data. Finally, record review is labor-intensive, involving hours of reading.

Self-Report Diary

A self-report diary is a self-monitoring technique that has been widely used in health promotion programs, especially for smoking cessation and weight control. Participants are given a diary in which to record and monitor a target behavior over a period of time. Both the participant and evaluator can identify and track knowledge and behavioral change recorded in the participant's own words. This opportunity for self-awareness and insight distinguishes diaries from other data collection methods. Diaries may be qualitative or quantitative in nature.

The diary method has also been applied to HIV/AIDS prevention. It has been used in at least three different prevention programs targeted at gay men (Gordon, 1987; Kelly & St. Lawrence, 1988; Mantell, DiVittis, Kochems, & Ostfield, 1989b) for self-monitoring of sexual activities. These diaries had structured questions that made it easier for participants to identify triggers to high-risk activities and comply with daily or weekly recording requirements. The responses to these questions, however, were open-ended. Participants recorded such activities as: (1) nature and frequency of their sexual activities; (2) events that took place immediately prior to high-risk sexual activity; (3) the social context in which sexual behavior occurred (e.g., the setting in which the risky behavior took place, use of alcohol and/or drugs preceding the event, mood, cognitive intentions prior to the sexual encounter, and sexual fantasies that preceded or took place afterward); and (4) sexual and sensual goals for physically and emotionally safer sex. An example of a section of a diary regarding sexual behavior that is primarily qualitative with open-ended responses about sexual encounters (and a few questions with close-ended responses) is presented in Example 7.2.

This same strategy can be used to characterize other HIV risk behaviors, such as alcohol and drug use. The diary is an ideal means for capturing wellness activities such as exercise and nutrition.

The use of diaries as a data collection method has several benefits. In monitoring a behavior on a daily basis, the behavior is documented close to the time when it happened. This should presumably strengthen participants' recall ability, and therefore increase reliability of the data gathered with this method. Further, because such assignments are

---

Example 7.2. Selected Section from Self-Report Sexual Behavior Diary

Have you had a sexual experience of any kind this week? [ ] Yes [ ] No
If YES ↓
How many? _____
How many of them were with other people? _____
How many different people? _____

Think about any one of these sexual encounters. In the space below, write about it. Include such things as: Where were you before you had sex? What were you doing? How were you feeling before you had sex? Were any substances involved (e.g., alcohol or pot)? Did you find the experience satisfying? Did you know your partner well? Was the experience low risk in terms of HIV transmission? What, if anything, would you have changed about this experience (e.g., could it have been safer?)

(SOURCE: Mantell *et al.*, 1989a.)

---

often novel to the participants, compliance at the onset of data collection is usually high. Their pencil-and-paper, self-monitoring procedures make diaries easy to administer and inexpensive.

Diaries incorporated into an intervention can engage clients, giving them a sense of empowerment as active participants in their behavioral change process. For families who set their own goals for problem-solving and coping with AIDS, diaries record goal-setting and its attainment. The consequence is that the assessment tool, while designed to evaluate, becomes an intervention in itself, capable of influencing the participants' knowledge, attitudes, and behavior. Monitoring the behavior can be a powerful behavior modification tool, serving to deter adoption of unhealthy activities. These recordings become meaningful to the evaluators as well as the participants. Diary information can be a catalyst for the development of new risk-reduction interventions.

Disadvantages of Method

Some weaknesses of the diary method include:

- Labor intensity for investigator throughout the data collection and analysis phases.
- Difficulty in controlling the consistency of participants' reporting patterns.
- Participants' fear that the diary will be discovered by others.
- Distortion of data through participants' efforts to present themselves in the most positive, or socially desirable, light; therefore, recorded behavior may not reflect actual behavior.
- Lack of compliance among those who do not write well or are embarrassed about their writing; therefore, the diary method may be unsuitable for use with low-literate and illiterate populations. Effectively, this method could not be used with many subsets of the population most at risk for HIV who tend to have limited education.
- Decline over time in participant interest and compliance.

When there is a choice of evaluation methods, a problem frequently encountered is that the participants' preferred method is not the most efficacious one for collecting data. For example, one study of gay male prostitutes indicated that their recall of high-risk sexual behaviors was better with a self-administered instrument than with a diary; however, 86% of the sample preferred the diary recording to the self-administered questionnaire (McLaws *et al.*, 1990).

Vignettes

A vignette is another data collection method that may be qualitative or quantitative in nature, depending on whether response choices are predetermined or open-ended. Vignettes tell a story in which hypothetical dilemmas based on descriptions of real-life situations are posed and resolved by participants. The solution is not presented; rather, the participant is asked to solve the problem or complete the story. Sexual behavior (e.g., condom negotiations), gender scripting (e.g., which partner has responsibility for assuring that condoms are used), drug use (e.g., refusal of injecting or sharing equipment), household decision-making (e.g., renting an apartment, child care), and disclosure of HIV status (e.g., telling partner only, family only, or no one) are domains that could be tapped in these vignettes. Based on the solutions suggested, participants' competency can be self-rated, rated by their partners, or by trained observers or judges using videotapes.

Vignettes can be used to assess program impact, for example, in terms of participants' cognitive problem-solving competency (Spivak, Platt, & Shure, 1976; Goldfried & D'Zurilla, 1969) and assertiveness skills development in relation to specific target behaviors (Phillips, 1985; Curran, 1985). Problem-solving skills include problem identification, goal-setting, alternative thinking, anticipation of obstacles, resource identification, and means–ends planning (i.e., developing strategies for goal attainment).

Vignettes are effective cross-validation tools when used in combination with other evaluation methods, such as personal interviews, diaries or logs, behavioral role-plays, and taped dyadic interaction records. Information from these vignettes can be compared with structured interview data to identify areas of inconsistency, e.g., discrepancies in condom use.

Disadvantages of Method

One problem with the use of vignettes is that the evaluator does not know how the participant will react to these dramas. Without understanding the situations of individual respondents, the evaluator needs to be trained to manage a variety of reactions, some of which may be highly emotional due to the subject matter.

Observational Measures

Direct observation of behaviors is another technique that is qualitative when the observations are not recorded into a highly structured closed-ended format (e.g., checklists, multiple choice). Observation entails watching and listening to things said by the people being studied over some period of time, the exact form of which may vary. Participant interactions, rituals, routines, and social organization are typically recorded, supplemented by a description of participants' appearance, roles, and entrances and exits in the observed setting (Adler & Adler, 1994). These observations are recorded in field notes. There is no one way to record. Some recordings will be free thought associations in a notebook; in other cases, recording will be more structured, depending on the purpose of the data collection.

Observational techniques can be used as part of a strategy to recruit subjects. The observation of STD clinic operations prior to recruiting a sample of women can aid the evaluator in identifying means of enrolling participants into a preventive intervention. Knowledge of attendance patterns and patient flow can help the evaluator to identify optimal days and times for recruitment so as to maximize program enrollment. For example, if observational data reveal that the average waiting time before seeing a clinician is more than an hour, the evaluator can capitalize on this "down" time and screen women to ensure that they meet the eligibility criteria for program participation.

Direct observation of behavior is also used in process evaluation. For example, to assess whether a program is being implemented according to plan, trained observers may be randomly assigned to observe program activities and interactions between the group facilitator and participants.

Observation is also useful for learning about the behavior of two people (a dyad) or a larger group. For example, observing dyadic interactions in relation to sexual negotiations and decision-making is an important but underutilized technique in understanding women's and men's precautionary sexual behavior. An interactional sequence can be videotaped. Observation and coding of a videotaped interactional sequence among heterosexual couples can be used to assess how partners in both new and long-term relationships negotiate for safer sex and resolve conflicts, and to compare similarities and differences in strategies between male and female partners and by types of partnership.

Disadvantages of Method

The main criticisms leveled against observational methods relate to their reliability and validity, since interpretation is subjective, relying on the observer's perceptions. The observer unknowingly may view events and behaviors selectively. The use of multiple observers to "rate" the same sequence of events and behaviors can alleviate this problem, however. Participant observation, in which the researcher goes "native" and integrates him or herself into the study subjects' setting, poses potential problems for the observer–researcher. If the observer discloses to participants his or her role as a researcher, he or she can influence the individual or community being observed. Alternatively, a researcher's failure to disclose his or her role as observer might be perceived as unethical (Babbie, 1973). Other limitations of observational methods include the inability to view and record each event as it happens and the use of non-systematic techniques (Babbie, 1973).

Ethnographic Methods

Ethnographic approaches to qualitative evaluation research, traditionally used by anthropologists, are characterized by three distinct features: (1) prolonged contact with a community; (2) concern for day-to-day events; and (3) direct or indirect participation in local activities (Miles & Huberman, 1994). Atkinson and Hammersley (1994) refer to ethnography as not only a method, but a philosophical orientation. Other common features of ethnographic research, many of which are also core characteristics of the qualitative paradigm, according to Atkinson and Hammersley (1994), are:

- Emphasis on exploration of social phenomena.
- Work with unstructured (uncoded) data.
- Investigation of a small number of cases.
- Interpretation of the meanings and functions of human behavior, primarily in the form of verbal descriptions and explanations.

Ethnographic methods may be used for evaluation, as a monitoring tool, and for an intervention. Multiple sources of data collection are typically used, including participant and structured nonparticipant (indirect) observation, in-depth unstructured interviews, case study, archival documents, diary review, videotaping, and oral histories. Regardless of the purpose of the ethnography, these methods must be applied systematically.

Following the completion of an in-depth ethnographic study, quantitative data collection methods, e.g., a survey of community members' drug use and injection practices, are frequently used to interpret qualitative findings.

As with other qualitative methods, human behavior is reconstructed within the cultural and social context where it occurs (Spradley & McCurdy, 1972; Spradley, 1979). As a result of extended contact, an evaluator can acquire firsthand, from the respondents' point of view, an in-depth understanding of the traditions of a target group or community. The intent is to reduce social distance and improve rapport between people of different worlds—the researcher and the group or population under study (Agar, 1986).

Altheide and Johnson (1994) suggest nine essential dimensions to be covered in ethnographic field notes and reports about a population or community:

- Historical, physical, and environmental contexts.
- Number of participants and key informants.
- Range of activities.
- Origins and consequences of significant events in participants' lives.
- Temporal order of events.
- Division of labor and hierarchies.
- Patterns of routines and their variations.
- Participants' perspectives and meanings of accounts.
- Social rules, codes, and patterns of order.

The ethnographic method serves a number of functions in the evaluation and ongoing monitoring of HIV prevention programs. It is particularly proficient for eliciting information about behaviors perceived to be taboo, such as anal sex and male-to-male or female-to-female sex; or illegal, such as injecting drugs or trading sex for money, drugs, or shelter (Schensul & Schensul, 1990). These methods allow evaluators to observe persons in their daily lives regularly and create a climate of tolerance and candor that encourages participants to share intimate information in their own words and time.

In addition, this approach is useful for studying populations that are frequently difficult for professionals to reach. To gain access to a "hidden" high-risk population such as lesbian injection drug users, community service sites for the lesbians and injection drug users can be canvassed. For example, one San Francisco study identified bars, street corners, and neighborhoods where lesbian injection drug users could be found (Case, Downing, Fergusson, Lorvick, & Sanchez, 1988). This is called cataloguing the community or ethnographic mapping. Outreach workers then used three methods to recruit participants into the study: (1) "chain referral" or "snowball" sampling (subjects' recommendation of other people for the researcher to contact); (2) placement of posters where lesbian injection drug users tended to congregate; and (3) referrals from other studies.

In the following sections, we describe three facets of an in-depth ethnographic approach: (1) direct observation, (2) rapid assessment, and (3) intervention.

Direct Observation

The predominant qualitative technique used in ethnographic research to gain greater understanding of a community is direct observation. These observations take place within the context of a naturalistic setting, where the observation follows the natural sequence of events. Observers do not ask research questions or lead a focus group; active participation of community members is not required. Rather, the observers' role is to watch participants in a group or an area of a community. However, following a more contemporary perspective, some researchers have achieved a different balance of involvement—adopting roles of complete-member–researcher, active-member–researcher, and peripheral-member–researcher in these naturalistic settings (Adler & Adler, 1994).

Information about a community's beliefs, values, norms, behaviors, and hidden codes of conduct is essential to the planning, design, and content of culturally sensitive HIV preventive interventions. For example, in-depth investigation of levels of transculturation (i.e., the ability of a non-US-born individual to adopt sociocultural norms and values of the dominant culture and, at the same time, to influence the dominant culture) (Ortíz-Torres, Rapkin, Mantell, & Tross, 1992); gender-role beliefs and behavior related to sexuality, contraception, and pregnancy; and the social context of community life (e.g., language, community size, socioeconomic status, age distribution, and violence) may be especially important.

When observing community members within their environment, the evaluator is particularly interested in identifying the gatekeepers and institutions through which the community can be reached (e.g., churches, organizations, and hangouts). Observations after an intervention can also provide information on various changes resulting from program participation. If, for example, one of a program's goals is to create an atmosphere where safer sex practices can become normative, observation of a community member's behavior in that setting could well provide an example of just such changes. The relatively prolonged time period required for observation, the need for highly skilled observers, and labor-intensive data analysis make this technique expensive.

Rapid Ethnographic Assessment Inventory

Traditional ethnographic methods such as direct observation require a long period of time for scrutiny and may involve living within the study community. The Rapid Ethnographic Assessment Inventory (REAI), developed by the World Health Organization's Global Programme on AIDS (Scrimshaw, Carballo, Ramos, & Blair, 1991), is a practical technique for establishing a quick and detailed cultural profile of a community. It focuses on a few topics in a short period of time and is particularly useful for AIDS projects with limited resources for intervention. Although most effective for formative evaluation, this technique can be employed throughout multiple phases of research such as in program design, implementation, maintenance, and replication.

REAI incorporates a number of research methodologies: formal and informal interviews, conversation, direct observation and participant observation, personal diaries, and secondary sources of data collection. Combining quantitative survey instruments with a period of observation can help minimize the potential discrepancy between reported and actual behaviors.

The REAI technique is helpful in understanding a group's beliefs about AIDS and motivations for practicing high-risk behavior. The results from these assessments are

Careful thought needs to be given to whether a focus group is the best method for obtaining the desired information. If the topics are sensitive, group interaction might inhibit the truth or participants from sharing ideas. Under such circumstances, an individual questionnaire or face-to-face interview might be a better choice. If a researcher wants to understand why a particular program succeeded or failed, then a focus group may be the most effective and rapid method of information retrieval.

Selecting Participants: Group Structure and Composition. The focus group is usually comprised of a small number of volunteer participants (no fewer than 6 and no more than 12) solicited from the target group (e.g., the community) through media advertisements or participation in existing organizations or classes. As part of the recruitment process, participants should be informed about the interview topic(s). To minimize sampling bias, group participants should be chosen to reflect specific segments of the target population of interest. Usually it is preferable to select participants who do not know each other, since familiarity might inhibit group discussion.

Group composition is typically sociodemographically homogeneous. However, sometimes groups are sociodemographically mixed. The choice will depend on the objective of the information base and the topics to be covered. For instance, homogeneous groups should be similar to one another in ways that are relevant to the topic, so members can interact in a meaningful manner. If the purpose of the focus group is to examine the relationship between gender-role norms and sexual behavior, the researcher may want to include both women and men in the group. (However, separate same-gender groups could be conducted.) If the focus group is targeted to adolescent girls and the topic is condom negotiation skills to prevent HIV infection, then participants should all have the same status, e.g., being single or in a partnered relationship. Variables the evaluator might want to match in selecting group participants are cultural background, social class, age, and experience. Convening two or three groups helps to assure that there is a range of participants represented in the larger population through age, sociopolitical, and economic background.

Convening Focus Groups: The Importance of the Physical Environment. The physical site of the focus groups should be inviting, easily accessible by private or public transportation, safe, temperature controlled, and with enough lighting to enable participants to see one another. Freedom from interruption and privacy must also be ensured to facilitate participation. Providing refreshments can be an incentive to participation and can serve as a prop, helping group members to relax.

The moderators' roles. Groups are led by a trained moderator who is gentle, friendly, and able to engage participants in a discussion based on guided questions. Often there is a need for more than one moderator. The moderator should be someone who speaks the native language and who is familiar with the community and its culture. The moderator must also be trained in how to facilitate group discussion, since he or she aims to stimulate discussion among group members rather than one-way facilitator–participant interactions. Level of moderator involvement may vary, ranging from nondirective to a rigid control of topic choice and interaction between group members. The more specific the type of information needed, the more directive the moderator needs to be. If group members ask a lot of questions, the moderator should defer giving information until the end of the formal group discussion.

When members do not participate in the discussion, the moderator should encourage them to share their views. At the same time, the moderator should ensure that particular group members do not dominate the discussion or continually interrupt others. The moderator regulates the physical and psychological environment of the setting, ensuring that it is intimate, nonthreatening, and promotes candid communication (Basch, 1987).

The moderator should begin the group with introductions of self and participants. As part of this "icebreaker," participants can be asked to state their reasons for participating in the group. Ground rules, e.g., confidentiality (what is discussed in the group should not be shared with nongroup members), that every member's participation is important, or that there are no correct or incorrect responses with regard to personal beliefs and experiences, should be stated prior to discussing the group topic.

Monitoring of group interaction. Activities are monitored via audio tape and/or by direct observation by one or more individuals. Observers should listen carefully to the group discussion, monitor nonverbal cues, and avoid projecting their own values and interpretations onto the participants. These observers should sit outside the group so as to minimize their distracting participants. Notes from these observations are then recorded and transcribed. Participants can also be recorded through one-way mirror observation or audio- or videotaping. Participants are often not referred to by their full name; rather, first names or pseudonyms may be used to protect their identities. It is essential to let participants know they will be recorded or observed as well as to obtain a signed informed consent.

Developing and using an interview guide. The research team and/or facilitator prepares a list of topic areas ranging from the general to the specific. Each question needs to be tied to eliciting particular types of information so that the interview remains focused. To keep the session evenly paced, a time schedule for responses to these questions should be generated in advance. Because there is always potential for participants to be reluctant to discuss a particular topic area or question, a list of probing questions to encourage communication should be developed for each topic area. Probes can also be prepared impromptu during the group session, such as paraphrasing what participants have said, asking for details, and challenging group members.

Reviewing the data for report preparation. The moderator, recorder, and observer should compare impressions immediately following the focus group. Reviewing the tapes and constructing the report can be done by the moderator alone or in conjunction with other members of the research team. A summary of the steps involved in conducting a focus group are described in Table 7.6.

Advantages of Method. Focus groups offer both participants and evaluators many benefits. Through participant selection, this technique empowers the individual to see him or herself as an "expert," while providing the opportunity to share ideas with similar people who are sought out for their opinions. During the group, people can participate when they feel they have something to contribute or can remain silent on issues. Group interviewing is a synergistic or combined group effort that produces a wider range of

Table 7.6. Steps in Conducting a Focus Group[a]

The focus group is a discussion of predetermined content areas that lasts from 1 to 2 hours. The steps in conducting the groups are:

- Warm up: Beginning with introductions can make participants more comfortable. An innocuous question can also be an "ice-breaker," helping to make participants feel at ease.
- Norms and roles: It is essential to describe the role of the facilitator as someone who moves the discussion along, makes sure that all persons have the chance to participate, and does not interject his/her personal opinions. Confidentiality of all responses is assured and recording techniques are explained. Participants are told there are no right or wrong answers and the facilitator will not judge responses.
- General to specific: Discussions move from general to specific. Closing questions are often related to specific program suggestions or products.
- Open-ended probes: All questions are open-ended. If there are no responses or they are limited, phrases to encourage discussion can be used to elicit more discussion.
- Recording for posterity: Although it requires equipment and personnel, tape recording is most effective to document what was said. Augmentation through observers helps to record facial expressions and body language as well as physical location of participants.

[a]From Runkle (1990).

information, insights, and ideas than individual interviews. Answers to the structured questions can have a "snowball" effect, where one comment spontaneously leads to another.

Disadvantages of Method. Despite the multiple advantages of focus groups, they have several limitations. These include: (1) difficulty in moderating the group; (2) difficulty in interpretation and in drawing firm conclusions (Bellenger, Bernhardt, & Goldstucker, 1976); (3) potential high costs of recruiting and paying group members; (4) limited generalizability due to nonrepresentative samples; (5) potential biased interpretation of recorded transcripts (Basch, 1987); and (7) dependence on the facilitator's skills.

Different Applications of Focus Groups. A focus group is an excellent mechanism to provide direction on how to proceed with program development. Feedback from focus groups supplies background information, which helps the researcher to: (1) assess the needs of the target population; (2) explore new program ideas, shape intervention content, and determine implementation strategy; and (3) identify messages for risk-reduction/prevention materials, understand the vocabulary and assumptions about specific topics, e.g., sex or birth control, develop questions for structured interviews, and generate hypotheses. Eight applications of focus groups, and specific examples of these applications are discussed below:

1. *Identify needs of a target audience and barriers to service.* Staff of a family planning program believed adolescent males to be the "missing link" in the prevention of unintended pregnancies and STDs (Knox, Rhoades, & Deatrick, 1988). Focus groups and client satisfaction surveys were used to determine adolescent males' need for sexuality education and reproductive health services. Fifty-three adolescent males participated in six focus group sessions, and six structured interviews were held with individuals and couples. The groups convened for 90-minute sessions, with five to nine

males attending each session. Scenarios were constructed to obtain participant reactions to contraception and sexual responsibility.

Results of the focus group and individual interviews indicated that adolescent males, despite a high demand for sexuality/contraceptive education, perceived barriers to receiving such education. Barriers that inhibited their access to clinical services, such as embarrassment in discussing sexual issues, were viewed as high. Negative feelings about condom use were associated with embarrassment in purchasing them, decreased sensation, and fear of breakage. While the positive aspects of condom use—that they are "smart" to use, prevent pregnancy and STDs, and are readily accessible—were mentioned, participants perceived the negative aspects to far outweigh the positive. The focus groups also revealed gender differences: adolescent males wanted programs to be more interactive and less didactic and preferred coeducational to same-sex programs. Skills development (particularly in the area of communication), opportunities to discuss emotional aspects of contraceptive use, and relationships were all cited as important.

Thus, these focus group data provided valuable, detailed information about the content of pregnancy and STD prevention programs and also underscored the need to engage males in family planning services.

2. *Guide program content.* The researcher or HIV/AIDS educator can apply focus group methods to develop the content of an intervention. The scenarios for role plays, the use of exercises, and the scope of presentation content can be guided by focus group findings. Sikkema, Winett, and Lombard (1995a) used a series of focus groups to identify role-play situations that could be used in the assessment of sexual assertiveness skills and intervention among college-aged women.

Through these group discussions, the researchers learned that this group of college students were knowledgeable about general AIDS information. Based on these data, a more specific measure of AIDS knowledge, which tapped STD and risk behavior management and social norms, was constructed. Learning that women in long-term relationships of 3 to 4 years did not report high-risk behaviors enabled the researchers to exclude this subgroup from the intervention.

A second series of focus groups were conducted with ten heterosexual male college students to shed light on their attitudes about increasing women's sexual assertiveness. The data indicated that the men's knowledge, attitudes, and behaviors were similar to those of the women. In addition, the men generally endorsed the notion of women being sexually assertive.

These findings were then applied to develop role-play scenarios for the intervention. The scenarios related to alcohol use, sexual encounters with a new partner, a sexually active relationship in which the woman takes birth control pills, and a male friend, who was feeling down.

3. *Develop HIV prevention messages.* Focus groups can also be helpful in developing appropriate messages for public service announcements for specific target populations, such as women, injection drug users, gay and bisexual men, African Americans, Latinos, Asians, Native Americans, adolescents, and migrant laborers. In the case of a public service announcement campaign directed to adolescents, focus groups can identify what kinds of language will be appropriate for that group, pinpoint their

beliefs about the availability and acceptability of condom use, and identify motivators for behavioral change (Winett *et al.*, 1990).

Similarly, focus groups can be used to develop age-appropriate and culturally competent prevention messages for media campaigns. Using focus groups in a series of multifaceted workshops for youth in Soweto, South Africa, Parker (1995) was able to empower the group to develop prevention messages for teens by teens. At the end of the 3- to 4-hour workshops, the group of teens produced three posters, four radio spots, and a range of slogans. The next step in the research process is to evaluate the acceptability and impact of these prevention media on the target audience.

4. *Assess appropriateness of prevention materials for target audience.* A target audience's reactions to an AIDS prevention video, brochure, or media campaign can be determined with focus group interviews. By identifying cultural values and social norms about AIDS and related risk behaviors, these interviews can be used to fine-tune the cultural specificity of HIV prevention information materials. For example, with an inner-city Latino population, focus group findings might reveal strong cultural values, such as discomfort in talking about sex in mixed company, male authoritarianism, protection of one's family, the family as caregiver, and the preservation of fertility. Learning that HIV prevention behaviors, e.g., condom use, are inconsistent with group values should alert the evaluator to the need for reframing the program's messages to be consistent with group norms.

To develop a better condom distribution brochure, the San Francisco AIDS Foundation conducted a focus group with male and female sex workers. Information from these interviews was used to modify the educational material so that it would be more effective for the intended audience. Discussion centered on the impact of AIDS on their lives, sources of AIDS information, knowledge and behavior regarding condom use, spermicides, injecting drugs, and cleaning "works."

Another example of using focus groups for material development was work done by the New York City Department of Health's Women and AIDS Committee (Duke *et al.*, 1989). Nine focus groups, composed of women (and in some cases, men) representative of diverse New York City target groups, were conducted to determine reactions to various sections of a draft version of a *Women and AIDS* brochure. The focus groups were intended to assess the clarity, accuracy, responsiveness, and sensitivity of the brochure. The nine groups were chosen for the diversity of member characteristics and included women in methadone maintenance and drug-free treatment, HIV-infected men and women, foster mothers/caretakers, clients of community-based organizations, homeless women, lesbians, and community service providers. The questionnaire that guided the group sessions and comments from group members is presented in Table 7.7.

5. *Determine perceptions of HIV infection in a community.* Focus groups can be helpful in determining a community's level of AIDS awareness and how it has been affected by the disease, as well as its prevalence of high-risk behaviors and attitudes toward the messages and channels of communication used to reach that community. To learn what women knew and thought about HIV/AIDS testing and partner notification, the New York City Department of Health conducted ten focus groups with diverse groups of women, e.g., patients in a health center, members of the Junior League, clients in drug

Table 7.7. Focus Group Questions and Comments
to Evaluate a Women and AIDS Brochure[a]

Questions

- Did you understand the information?
- Was the information stated clearly? If not, how would you make it clearer?
- Is the information presented in a logical sequence? Are there any words you did not understand? Is the information accurate?
- Is any of the information offensive to you? Why? How would you change it?
- Is there anything you especially liked? Disliked? What/why?
- Is there anything that you would change?

- Do you think that women will find this information useful?
- Would you pick this up and read it if you saw it in a clinic or doctor's office?
- Having read this brochure, would you show it to a friend?
- Do you have any suggestions of where this brochure can be distributed so that women will have access to it?
- Is this brochure designed for you?
- How does this brochure affect you?
- What should have been covered that wasn't?

Comments of focus group members

- "Should always state drugs, *including alcohol*."
- "Why is alcohol a risk for AIDS?"
- "How can you get AIDS from crack?"
- "The stuff about Crisco and Vaseline was weird!"
- "Add warning that some packaged needles on the street are *not* new, and don't use a needle that isn't in a sealed package."
- "Emphasize in big letters, bold and underlined, that you can't tell if someone is infected by the way they look. That is so important. I used to think you could tell. He *looked* clean, and now I'm infected."

- "If condom graphics are used in the brochure, emphasis should be put on pulling out before ejaculation."
- "I agree with the part against douching. Our vagina is like a self-cleaning oven. We don't need to douche."
- "Add that using a diaphragm does not protect you from AIDS."
- "Add that lambskin condoms are the same as animal skin condoms, and explain why we shouldn't use them (e.g., they are porous and the virus can pass through them)."

[a]From Duke *et al.* (1989).

treatment, and adolescents (Mantell, 1990). Table 7.8 presents an interview guide for a series of focus groups regarding community knowledge about HIV/AIDS transmission, prevention, testing, and partner notification. Information from these focus groups provided the New York City Department of Health with pertinent information about community knowledge and attitudes about HIV, testing, and partner notification to inform the development of their HIV programs and policies.

    6. *Develop and refine assessment tools.* Focus groups are particularly useful to develop content for questionnaires/interviews and assure that they are culturally and linguistically appropriate. For example, in a study of couples' HIV beliefs and intentions, focus groups can be used to refine a structured assessment of divergent HIV intentions and sexual negotiation and decision-making processes. Thus, to develop closed-ended questions for a structured interview, focus groups can be conducted with a representative sample of the target population to identify salient behavioral beliefs underlying behavioral performance and referents for normative measures. For example, to identify salient outcomes associated with a man's use of condoms during vaginal sex, the questions

Table 7.8. Excerpts from Interview Guide
for Focus Groups re: Beliefs about HIV/AIDS[a]

General

   1. What are some of the things you've heard about how people get AIDS?
   2. Do you know anyone who has AIDS or is infected with HIV? If yes, how has this affected you?
   3. Do you think you could tell if you had HIV? If yes, how? If no, why not?
   4. Do you think you could get AIDS? If yes, how? If no, why not?
   5. If someone is HIV-infected, what can be done for him/her medically?

Prevention

   6. If you thought your girlfriend was at risk, what would you tell her about how to protect herself from getting infected with HIV?

Knowledge

   7. What are some things you can do to protect yourself from getting AIDS?

HIV Testing

   8. What have you heard about the HIV test?
   9. How important is it to know if you have HIV?
  10. Is there a particular clinic, health center, doctor's office, or other place you usually go to if you are sick or need advice about your health?
  11. What types of tests do you think are done when you have your blood drawn?
  12. What does it mean if your doctor doesn't say anything to you about the AIDS virus?
  13. What would make you want to get tested for HIV? What would stop you from getting tested?
  14. If you got tested, who would you tell about your test results? How would you feel if you had to tell someone that you had HIV? What types of reactions do you think you would get?
  15. Is it important for you to ask your partner to be tested?
  16. What would you do if your partner asked you to be tested?

Partner Notification

  17. Have you ever been notified by the Health Department about being exposed to a STD? If yes, what was it like for you?
  18. If one of your partners tested positive for HIV and the Health Department told you, what would that be like for you?
  19. What do you think happens to the names given to the Health Department for notification of exposure to a STD or HIV?
  20. What do you think would happen if the Health Department told your sex partner(s) that you had tested HIV-positive?

[a]From Mantell (1990).

regarding his main sexual partner and social network members listed in Example 7.3 could be posed. A content analysis of responses to these questions is conducted to identify the most frequently mentioned outcomes and salient referents.

   7. *Validation of instruments.* The focus group format can be used to assess how well the instrumentation of an intervention measures the desired constructs. Through group discussion, participants are asked for their impression of the meaning of items in a given questionnaire. This is a form of content validity, where the focus group serves as a "panel of experts." Their feedback is used by the researcher to determine the appropriateness of item wording and meaning and to make any modifications in instrumentation.

   8. *Improve subject receptivity and responsiveness to the research program.* Finally, designs and recruitment procedures can be enhanced by focus group data. Such information can increase the evaluation researcher's understanding of the target population and ultimately lead to improved subject participation and retention rates.

Example 7.3. Focus Group Guide to Determine Salient Outcomes Associated with Condom Use from Male Perspective

---

Questions

- What do you see as the advantages (positive outcomes of, benefits of, good things that would happen) of your always using a condom for vaginal sex with your main sexual partner?
- What do you see as the disadvantages (negative outcomes, costs, bad things that would happen) of your always using a condom for vaginal sex with your main sexual partner?
- What else comes to mind when you think about always using a condom for vaginal sex with your main sexual partner? For example, how would always using a condom for vaginal sex with your main sexual partner make you feel? How would it make others feel? How would they react?

Relevant Referents (Perceived Sources of Social Influence/Normative Pressure)

- List those individuals or groups who would support or approve of your always using a condom for vaginal sex with your main sexual partner.
- List those individuals or groups who would oppose or disapprove of your always using a condom for vaginal sex with your main sexual partner.
- List any other individuals or groups that come to mind when you think about always using a condom for vaginal sex with your main sexual partner.

(SOURCE: Fishbein *et al.*, 1991.)

The initiation of a perinatal HIV prevention program in the women's clinics of a metropolitan New York City hospital illustrates how a focus group can facilitate acceptance by an organization. A series of focus groups were conducted with staff at varying levels at a hospital targeted to receive an intervention program to reduce HIV transmission among female patients. The goals of the focus group were to invest the staff in the program and facilitate the hospital's acceptance of the program. The overall theme of the group was to elicit provider feedback that, when appropriate, would be included in the program. Example 7.4 contains a segment of the focus group questions posed to staff.

MANAGING AND ANALYZING QUALITATIVE DATA

Management and analysis of qualitative data, like quantitative data management and analysis, is not a haphazard process. Though the qualitative approach entails semistructured and unstructured questions that yield open-ended responses, systematic standardized procedures have been developed to examine these data. Regardless of type of qualitative data collection method, analysis entails processing of written, taped, or filmed text in the form of field notes, observers' recordings, responses to open-ended

---

Example 7.4. Segment of a Focus Group for Staff
to Facilitate Acceptance of HIV Prevention Program

Program design
  Format
  Goal: To elicit feedback regarding logistical issues related to the setup of our intervention.
  Questions:
    How many sessions should we have?
    How long should each session be? Is a break needed?
    How often should we have these sessions?
    Where should these sessions be held? At what time?
    How large should each group be?
    How many groups do we want to have (i.e., how many participants do we want to recruit)?
  Goal: To determine the most appropriate method for presenting the material to participants.
  Question: What is the most effective format for presenting this material?

(SOURCE: DiVittis, Mantell, & Ramos, 1990b.)

---

questions, or audio- or videotaped scripts of interaction sequences or focus group discussions.

Using a grounded theory approach (Glaser & Strauss, 1967) to the data, the researcher begins with the initial hypotheses and concepts, but during the process of interacting with the data, may discard them, develop new guiding concepts, and test alternative hypotheses. Qualitative analysis is more likely to be an iterative process than the sequential approach of quantitative analysis. The major task is to explain how people account for the way they behave or think like they do within particular settings or situations. Data are first described and then analysis moves to a higher level of analytical abstraction to explain what is happening. The researcher searches for important ideas emerging and attempts to understand how they are linked. This is accomplished by looking at the regularities in behavior, patterns of events, and relationships among variables. Management of large volumes of field notes and narrative text data is maintained by such procedures as formatting the organization of data records, indexing and cross-referencing files (similar to procedures a librarian might institute to catalogue a library's collection of books and periodicals), summarizing the data, and establishing identifiers to retrieve data files.

Analytic Methods

In this section, we discuss two interactive components of qualitative data analysis: data reduction and data display, and draw heavily on the work of Miles and Huberman (1994).

Data Reduction

With qualitative data collection, the researcher often collects an abundance of data. To manage the vast amount of data and facilitate their interpretation, data reduction is necessary. Data reduction occurs continually throughout the project until the final report is written. Through coding, content analysis, and category and theme development, data reduction helps to focus analysis.

With quantitative data gathered from multiple choice or true–false questions, response categories are predetermined by the evaluator before the data are collected. Qualitative data, however, utilize open-ended or unstructured responses, reflecting the words of research participants. Observations are coded after they have been obtained. Content analysis essentially represents the assessment and aggregation of central thematic responses and scripts through coding procedures.

Coding.   Since texts from in-depth unstructured interviews or focus groups can be 50 pages or longer, the researcher needs to work with the data in a more manageable form. Coding is the primary technique for categorizing, summarizing, and reducing the data. Data reduction facilitates interpretation of the meaning of the data. Coding is an integral part of analysis, and it is the first step in preparing the data for further analysis. The researcher's ability to retrieve all text about a specific topic is then used to discover new insights about the data. Therefore, the ability to code and retrieve data is integral to its interpretation (Richards & Richards, 1994).

Identification of themes and exploration of meanings in the data demand a user-friendly system for coding the content of a narrative text and retrieving the coded text. This can be achieved with word processing or text search computer software programs that index coded sections of text, or with specially designed software for analyzing qualitative textual-level data. Revisions in codes are easier with computer systems. In the absence of accessibility to such technology, coding and analysis can also be done in the old-fashioned way—by hand. For example, some researchers use color codes when they cull through their field notes or transcribed narratives. This entails transferring the data to index cards and developing a coding system. Whatever method is used to organize the data, the ease of retrieval should be considered (Marshall & Rossman, 1995).

Coding Issues.   The researcher has to decide what units of information will be analyzed, i.e., what is to be coded. This might be a word, sentence, or paragraph, or in a couples' or focus group interview an exchange or discourse sequence. Another fundamental issue is how to assign meanings to observations or data collected, i.e., how does one observation differ from another, and the criteria to validate decisions in assigning these meanings, i.e., what are the codes.

The type of coding may vary, from simple descriptive codes, e.g., reflecting women's personal motivations for being tested for HIV, to codes that differentiate between motivations related to self versus those of partner, to those that are more inferential, e.g., grouping codes into a smaller set of units, themes, or constructs (Miles & Huberman, 1994). Codes should have some structural relationship to one another and not simply be a set of disjointed descriptive labels. What is important is that the codes have been clearly defined and operationalized so that multiple coders will apply the same rules and code a text in the same way. Another decision to be made is whether to assign multiple codes to a unit of analysis. The researcher must also determine what differences among observations are the most important to examine about a particular topic, i.e., prioritizing themes for in-depth analysis, and to whom these differences are important. Although labor-intensive, coding is necessary.

The researcher's dependence on particular theories and their assumptions will be made explicit in the development of a coding system. Hypotheses about the way in which coded variables relate to other measures and construct validity should be established.

The researcher also has to decide whether coding will be conducted within an individual or interpersonal context. Example 7.5 shows a coding scheme for patterns of negotiation styles related to condom use after the initial round of code development.

Both verbal and nonverbal behavior can be coded. In coding couples' interactions, the researcher has to decide whether to analyze each partner's responses independently (the individual response is the unit of analysis) and/or their joint responses (the couple and their interaction sequences are the units of analysis). Interaction sequences are then coded on the basis of a number of dimensions, which can be descriptive and/or evaluative.

Behavioral sequences can be segmented for quantification according to the principal act, inferred meaning of each interpersonal act, time, and events categories (Peterson, 1979; Schlundt & McFall, 1985). Peterson (1979) identified three criteria to evaluate these sequences: (1) a person's affect; (2) interpretation of messages, i.e., explaining the meaning of partner's and own behavior; and (3) expectation regarding partner's subsequent behavior. Although the data are qualitative, coding schemes are developed to aggregate or reduce the data into a more manageable form for interpretation.

Examples of other coding schemes that can be applied to quantify these interactional dialogues (Peterson, 1979; Schlundt & McFall, 1985) include:

- Emotions/affect (aggression; affiliation/approval; intimacy; sexual arousal; satisfaction/dissatisfaction with affect)

Example 7.5. Codes for Condom Negotiation Styles

- No discussion–no condom use
- Discussion that is misinformed, goes nowhere, or no decision is made
- No discussion–agreement to use condoms
- Not much talk, not much conflict, she tries different things and he doesn't care as long as it doesn't hassle him
- Conflict over condoms
- She is angry because he "screws up," e.g., he has no condoms available
- Negotiations in process
- History of open and egalitarian discussion with mutual support, openness to partners' influence whenever decisions come up

---

- Message/information content and its implications
- Adequacy of communication
- Asymmetrical/symmetrical initiation of questions
- Interrupted/completed statements
- Conversational control ("turns of talk")
- Style (interpersonal strategies and tactics employed: direct/indirect, active/ passive; verbal/nonverbal; behavioral demands)
- Normative rules
- Settling conditions—achieving resolution or consensus
- Outcome/consequences of the interaction (rewards and punishments for each party; effectiveness of influence)
- Use of problem-solving and conflict resolution strategies
- Extent of agreement or disagreement of partners' responses (i.e., concordance/ discordance)

Interrater judges are then used to assess the extent of judges' agreement with the initially coded sequences.

Procedures.   In preparation for analysis, data from focus groups, unstructured interviews, and open-ended questions from semistructured interviews should be transcribed verbatim. Following transcription, editing and correction of the audio- or videotapes will be required. Developing a recording system for documenting various levels of analysis is important. In reviewing narrative text, as suggested by Huberman and Miles (1994), researchers write analytic memos, i.e., written documentation, describing their thoughts on causal relationships between relevant concepts, surprising new findings, and intuitions about the validity of the data. Summaries of the setting in which the interviews/focus groups are conducted and descriptions of the participants are written. These analytic memos are then shared among the research team in study meetings to direct further analyses, coding systems for the primary constructs, and address possible problems in interpretation.

Transcripts of text are then reviewed and categorized by the researcher according to direct responses to questions and to themes that consistently emerge from the data. Coding is an ongoing process, with modifications made during the course of data collection after an initial set of codes is devised. This will allow the researcher to modify the interview guide. A preliminary coding system is developed and shared with all researchers. Content, context, and process are analyzed, initially described by simple one-word codes or abbreviations. As noted earlier, categorization is guided by the theoretical assumptions and framework of the research project.

A second coder should be used to code at least 10 pages of transcripts that have been analyzed by the first researcher (without having access to that researcher's remarks or coding) to ensure that most of the possible concepts are documented and explored. Disagreements and agreements should be recorded through analytic memos and discussed in research meetings. Interrater reliability (the number of agreements divided by the sum of agreements and disagreements) of the coding scheme is assessed through the calculation of the kappa coefficient. At the end of each data collection period, e.g., at the completion of the first of a series of three interviews, qualitative themes, constructs, and any linkages or discrepancies among them will be displayed in tabular form to facilitate further analysis.

Once this initial "pass" of the data is completed, using the agreed-upon coding scheme, all transcripts of tape-recorded focus groups and interviews need to be coded by the research team for content, process, relations among variables, contrasts and comparisons, frequency of patterns or events, and comparison to constructs already noted in the literature. New codes will inevitably arise as a result of this process and will have to be agreed upon by the research team (Huberman & Miles, 1994).

Interrater Reliability. The use of a systematic procedure for generating coding systems, coding the responses, and the calculation of interrater agreement of the codes will help to reduce bias due to the subjective perceptions of a single coder. This, in turn, should increase confidence in the validity, i.e., that the themes reflect what you believe they do, the reliability of the codes, and interpretation of the data. However, validity and reliability are also dependent on the judges having sufficient information and experience to make coding decisions. Sometimes, coding rules have to be refined so as to achieve adequate reliability.

The kappa statistic can be used to determine agreement among coders relative to that expected by chance. A negative value indicates less agreement than expected by chance when the relative prevalences of coding categories are taken into account, a 0 value indicates same agreement as expected, and a positive value indicates greater than expected agreement. A kappa coefficient of at least .7 is generally the criterion for agreement (Fleiss, 1973). In Table 7.9, we present an excerpt from the coding scheme and how five coders assigned codes for responses to an item tapping barriers to condom use among Puerto Rican men who have sex with men.

Table 7.9. Selected Response to an Open-Ended Question Tapping Barriers to Condom Use and Codes Assigned by Five Coders[a]

Responses	Coder 1	Coder 2	Coder 3	Coder 4	Coder 5
Sucking with a condom is less pleasurable	1B	1Ab	1Ab	1Ab	1D
El tenía un pene bello (He had a beautiful penis)	No code assigned	1Ab	1Ab	1Ab	5A

Selected coding scheme for opened-ended responses:

1. Respondents' pleasure	5. Lack of control
1A. Sensory	5A. Passion/arousal/excitement
a. Flesh-to-flesh	5B. Substance use
b. Other senses	5C. Impulsivity
1B. Interference with sexual function	
1C. Mood/romance	
1D. Dislike of condoms	

[a]From Psychosocial/Qualitative Assessment Core & Carballo-Diéguez (1994), with permission.

Analysis of Open-Ended Questions. When coding open-ended questions that are embedded in a structured interview, the same principles described above apply. Instead of pages of text, however, responses are limited to text of several sentences. Sometimes, the researcher may generate preliminary codes prior to administration of the interview to provide a first scan of the data, based on a theory-derived literature review. Additional codes can be generated based on either all of the responses or a random sample of a certain proportion of responses (depending on sample size). A question that elicits reasons for using a male or female condom with a set of predetermined codes is shown in Example 7.6.

When codes are not predetermined, the researcher must create a coding system from the observations, i.e., the coding scheme evolves from the data. For example, among women, in response to the question of "What do your intimate relationships mean to you?" the following issues should be addressed (Rapkin, 1995):

- What do you want to know about the ways in which women think and feel about their relationships with sexual partners?
- What type of language and terms do women use to connote these thoughts and feelings?

Example 7.6. Open-Ended Question with Set of Predetermined Codes

---

In the past 3 months, what led you to use male or female condoms *every time* you had intercourse? [WRITE ANSWER VERBATIM.]

[INTERVIEWER: CODE ABOVE ANSWER USING CODES BELOW. USE AS MANY AS NECESSARY]

Code list:

For protection against HIV/STDs
For pregnancy prevention
Wanted to try a new method—problems with other contraceptives
Wanted to try a new method—other reasons
Had an STD/partner had an STD
Temporary use (e.g., postpartum, postabortion, between methods)
New partner
Increased sense of risk/increased knowledge about HIV/STDs
Intervention
Influence of partner
Influence of friend
For protection, unspecified
Increased knowledge about method
Other
Missing/can't code

(SOURCE: Exner, Meyer-Bahlburg, Yingling, Hoffman, Ortíz-Torres, & Ehrhardt, 1993, with permission.)

- Can response categories be ordered? Are they mutually exclusive?
- Should responses elicited before interviewer probes be distinguished from those elicited after interviewer probes?
- Besides content, can any other information be gleaned from responses? (e.g., complexity, vagueness, distinction among partners versus generalization to all men?)

The process of codifying qualitative observations is a systematic and rigorous one. Table 7.10 elaborates a process for coding responses to open-ended questions.

Case Study: Assessment of Challenging Life Experiences. An analysis of open-ended questions in a semistructured interview of inner-city women related to barriers and facilitators to HIV testing serves as an example of how qualitative data can be reduced and analyzed into meaningful results. To develop a coding system for HIV/AIDS challenges faced by women, Enchautegui de Jesús, Rapkin, Mantell, Ortíz-Torres, and Tross (1996) used the responses of 300 women. One hundred and eighty (60%) of them contained accounts of challenging experiences.

Table 7.10. Steps for Developing a Coding Scheme
and Coding of Open-Ended Questions

1. Record verbatim each participant's response on a 5 × 8 index card or input the response into a computer file.
2. Reduce data by placing them in limited theme categories. (Initially a coder can be overwhelmed, as many themes may emerge.) If using index cards, sort them into piles according to broad themes emerging from the responses.
3. Multiple responses from a given participant should be coded and listed on separate cards.
4. Type a master list of themes and carefully review the piles of index cards for identification of subthemes. For example, if "self-esteem" is a major theme emerging from interviews with reproductive-age women, this category may be subdivided further into categories such as: "motherhood or pregnancy," "dependence on men," "perception of being nothing without a man."
5. Re-sort the original piles of index cards into new piles based on the refined categories and subcategories. The primary goal is to generate a coding scheme.
6. Convene a meeting of at least three but no more than five people, consisting of researchers as well as health educators and members of the target population. Formal academic training is not necessary to participate in this process.
7. The "lead" coder gives the coding team a list of the raw data (i.e., the verbatim responses of each participant) and the preliminary coding scheme developed by the lead coder and meets with them to discuss these codes. The goal of the meeting is to refine the original set of codes and reach consensus about a new coding scheme.
8. The coding team then uses the consensus coding scheme to code responses to the question.
9. A second meeting is convened to discuss how team members coded the responses. Based on this discussion and the problems that the coders had in applying the coding schemes, team members have the option of reconsidering and changing their codes. One hundred percent consensus is not essential, as the extent of consensus among coders will be assessed.
10. The extent of consensus among the coding team members, also called interrater reliability, is measured with the kappa statistic (which can be calculated on the computer with the *Statistical Package for the Social Sciences* program). This statistic should be reported in the final evaluation report or published journal article.

Coding system.   The development of the categories was based on both the data and a review of the literature on women and HIV, stress, coping, and social support. Twelve coding categories were developed by the researchers and then reviewed by other colleagues:

- Influence others to change or engage in a particular behavior.
- Resist pressure of others to engage in a certain behavior.
- Modify own values or beliefs, or confront social norms.
- Cope with economic hardship, overcome socioeconomic limitations, and/or pursue opportunities that improve her social or economic status.
- Deal with the actual or potential termination of an intimate relationship and its consequences.
- Cope with the actual or potential occurrence of abuse.
- Avoid or modify harmful behaviors or habits.
- Develop or demonstrate foresight.
- Cope with her own condition or illness and its consequences.
- Cope with parenting role and children-related situations.
- Cope with the death, illness, or potential uncontrollable loss of a significant other.
- Face a challenge different from those listed above.

Each response was also coded along six other dimensions (subcodes), when applicable:

- Who was involved in the challenge (e.g., partner, parent, child)?
- What specific behaviors or domains were entailed in the challenge (e.g., drug use, sexuality)?
- What was the valence of the challenge (i.e., positive or negative)?
- Was the challenge a reactive or a proactive one?
- What was the stage of the action or change (e.g., initiation, maintenance)?
- What were the consequences of the challenge (e.g., tangible, emotional)?

These dimensions captured the specific characteristics of the situations described by the participants in a structured and relevant way adequate for flexible data reduction.

The remaining open-ended questions in this section of the interview were content analyzed using 43 codes of specific helpful strategies or behaviors, 23 codes of unhelpful strategies, 19 for help received, and 15 for obstacles encountered. The codes emerged from actual responses and from pertinent classification schemes found in the literature (Marsella & Dash-Scheuer,1988; McCrae, Hill, St. John, Ambikapathy, & Garner, 1984; Menaghan, 1982; Nyamathi, Leake, Flaskerud, Lewis, & Bennett, 1993).

Data reduction strategy.   Every account of an experience was classified with one of the challenge codes described earlier and up to six subcodes, when appropriate. This level of detail was necessary to draw sound analogies to HIV prevention challenges. In developing these codes, the researchers strived for the greatest specificity so as to yield clearly interpretable and distinctive categories of experiences. However, decision rules to reduce the data were also based on the prevalence of the challenge codes and subcodes. Enough cases in each category to conduct adequate statistical analyses and a small number of categories to yield meaningful analyses were needed. The procedure to examine the data and explore data-reduction avenues entailed two steps: (1) obtaining summary statistics, and (2) conceptual interpretation of what would be meaningful categories based on the data-reduction guidelines described above.

The data describing the challenge were analyzed to explore the situational characteristics of the accounts offered and identify what categories of challenge could be developed for further statistical analysis. The prevalence of the different areas of challenges was assessed with frequency counts. A frequency count of each challenge dimension subcode was then obtained, which indicated whether there was variability along the different dimensions coded for each challenge account. Finally, cross-tabulation of the different dimensions allowed examination of how these dimensions converged. This analysis yielded seven categories of challenges considered to be prevalent and meaningful for analyzing competencies most relevant to HIV prevention and situationally distinctive in terms of stage of change, domain involved, or people involved. These categories were classified under two major themes. The first theme included behaviors directly analogous to HIV prevention: asserting one's desires or beliefs, quitting drug use, and deciding to terminate a relationship. The second theme was related to women's empowerment that may increase their ability to engage in preventive behaviors: improving living situation, overcoming income- and job-related difficulties, seeking educational opportunities, and being able to raise their own children.

Data Display

Data display refers to the visual presentation of the data. Just as a researcher in a quantitative study uses tables and figures to organize and present data in summary form, qualitative research findings should be distilled and presented in a systematic framework, e.g., the form of matrices (rows and columns on a table), charts, graphs, network linkages, summary of contacts with key informants, and reports of meetings regarding cases (Miles & Huberman, 1994). Displaying the data visually in some ordered fashion rather than relying solely on written text can help sharpen the focus of analysis. For example, the structure of an HIV-infected gay man's social network and the patterns of network members' endorsement for HIV prevention might be displayed in a chart. Matrices can be organized according to four elements: (1) descriptive or explanatory (describe what is versus what has occurred); (2) partially ordered or well-ordered (placement of data in rows and columns according to descriptive categories) versus some ordering (intensity of belief or behavior, participants' social roles); (3) time-ordered (looking at sequences and flow of the data); or (4) categories of variables (unit of analysis, specific acts or behaviors of the social units).

Four types of visual displays to describe data are common, according to Miles and Huberman (1994): (1) partially ordered (i.e., minimally ordered); (2) time-ordered (i.e., describe behavior in relation to flow of events); (3) role-ordered (i.e., interactions of people in their roles); and (4) conceptually ordered. In partially ordered displays, the researcher might map social network pathways for disseminating information about the female condom, the relationships among network members, and which members are positive about the method. Showing the number of people who sought HIV testing on a quarterly basis following Magic Johnson's public disclosure that he was HIV-positive is an example of a time-ordered data display. In a role matrix, the researcher might compare how familial support for HIV prevention differs according to roles (e.g., mother, father, spouse, children, or sibling). In a conceptually ordered display, for example, the barriers to introducing a hierarchy of female-controlled methods of HIV/STD prevention that give women a range of choices in STD and family planning clinics can be presented. These barriers might be reduced to two themes: providers' resistance to assuming additional job responsibilities, and providers' orientation toward prescription rather than encouraging client decision-making. In a matrix, the data would be organized according to problems associated with clinic organization and provider attitudes across the rows and strategies employed by the four sites across the columns. In noting patterns and themes, similarities and differences across variables and patterns of processes, i.e., how variables are connected across time and space within some context, can be identified. Clustering enables us to group concepts in order to conceptualize a phenomenon. Any combination of these types of displays can be used.

OTHER ISSUES IN DATA ANALYSIS

Three issues of concern related to data analysis are addressed below: (1) analysis of a single case versus multiple cases; (2) whether qualitative data should be quantified; and (3) analysis of focus group data.

Within-Case versus Cross-Case Analysis

A combination of both within-case and across-case analysis strategies can be employed to display and explain data. A detailed explanation of these issues can be found in Huberman and Miles (1994). Within-case analysis provides an account of what is going on with an individual case. It is a descriptive rendering—a story—of the sequences of events or interactions that took place. The full data are displayed and the researchers interact with the narrative text to develop explanations and reach conclusions about the data. A second focus of within-case analysis is to understand causal relationships among variables: how and why an event occurred. By looking at a temporal ordering of events over time within a case, the researcher attempts to explain how these events led to specific outcomes. For example, a researcher can look at the relationship among a man's attitudes about abortion, HIV-infected women bearing children, and whether a health department should notify the sex partners of an HIV-infected person. As another example, the relationship between stressful life events among drug users and their HIV risk behavior could be explored.

In contrast, cross-case analysis, the study of multiple cases, is a strategy that detects pattern clarification or "repeatable regularities" (Huberman & Miles, 1994). It determines whether the conceptual framework and patterns developed with the first case emerge in successive cases. The researcher is looking for similarities among respondents. These patterns may reflect recurring themes or configurations related to behaviors, social norms, and relationships across cases. For example, is there any pattern among women who say that they cannot convince their partners to use a condom? What do women who say they refuse to have sex with partners who will not use a condom have in common? How do these women differ from those who have unprotected sex because they are unable to convince their partners to use a condom? In this example, comparative analysis focuses on cases with different outcomes.

Distinct differences between subgroups may also be pursued. For example, the researcher could sift through the data to determine whether there are systematic response variations based on age, socioeconomic status, marital status, HIV risk behavior history, and ability to speak English. Looking for patterns across cases is analogous to the quantitative techniques of cluster analysis and factor analysis that seek to group data into smaller analytic units of common overarching themes, constructs, or profiles.

In addition to this case-oriented approach, an evaluator can use a variable-oriented analysis or an integration of the two approaches. In a variable-oriented analysis, the researcher looks for recurring themes or intercorrelations among variables that cut across cases, much the same way as in setting up a correlation matrix in quantitative research. This type of analysis is particularly useful for examining broad generalities in the data, but it is not able to deal effectively with complex causal relationships grounded in specific contexts (Miles & Huberman, 1994).

The study of multiple cases, particularly in multiple contexts or settings such as hospitals, drug treatment centers, and schools, can ensure that findings are not idiosyncratic, and thus increase their generalizability. Researchers often want to know whether their findings are applicable to similar populations in similar settings. Cross-case analysis also provides the researcher with a greater depth of understanding and explanation of the universal processes occurring across cases (Miles & Huberman, 1994).

Quantification of Qualitative Data

One issue that is often raised is the extent that it is appropriate to quantify qualitative data. Some researchers argue that submitting qualitative data to quantitative analysis defeats the purpose of qualitative methods, which aim to provide an in-depth exploration of a topic. This perspective is countered by those who believe that using terms such as "some," "most," or "few" to describe the number of respondents who adhere to a particular belief, norm, or behavior is imprecise. Our view is that the researcher needs to strike a balance on the qualitative–quantitative continuum, and that this should be propelled by the objectives of the research.

Tabulating the frequency of responses provides the researcher with an index of the range of responses, the majority and minority positions, and outliers. It also can give important information about changes over time, e.g., the trajectory of persons living with HIV. Numbers can allow the researcher to identify patterns among individuals with a particular characteristic, e.g., conservative attitudes about abortion among drug users. In addition, quantification can help verify hypotheses.

Analyses may consist of simple descriptive analyses that use numbers to rank the most salient themes and reflect the least-mentioned themes, count the number of times a person remarked about a particular theme, or rate the degree of some attitude across all cases. Indeed, as noted above, to establish the reliability of a coding system, qualitative observations are subjected to a quantitative index. As Miles and Huberman (1994) suggest, if you are going to transform qualitative data into quantities, these numbers should be presented in the context in which the data occur.

Analysis of Focus Group Data

The process and domains for coding focus group data are similar to those for coding interview text. The focus group interview is transcribed and analyzed for the range of responses, central themes, and shared perceptions, as well as dissenting or minority viewpoints. The meanings behind the spoken words are interpreted and the context of responses are documented. Major themes can be color coded to demarcate differences. The researcher may have to make several passes through the narrative text to delineate the multiple categories that emerged in the group discussion.

According to Stewart and Shamdasani (1990), content analysis of focus group interviews often addresses: (1) *importance*: what words, ideas, or symbols are consistently used (e.g., the number of times partner-related barriers to condom use is mentioned; (2) *direction or bias*: the relative distribution of favorable and unfavorable characterizations of a particular belief or symbol (e.g., the number of positive and negative characterizations regarding use of the female condom; and (3) *intensity of belief*: the kinds of qualifications and associations made in relation to a symbol or idea (e.g., the number of times female group members used emotionally charged words in relation to their male sexual partners).

Because the recorded narrative represents the conversation of a group rather than one individual, there are additional features to be considered. In determining the specific unit of information to analyze in focus group interviews, parts of the total group discussion are sampled. This is referred to as "sampling units" (Stewart & Shamdasani, 1990). The intent is to assure representative statements of the content of the group discussion.

The researcher also needs to develop rules for identifying relevant statements. For example, in coding responses to the theme of how gender roles influence HIV risk behavior among inner-city women, the following decisions need to be made (Rapkin, 1995):

- Will spontaneous statements or only direct responses in relation to probes be considered?
- Should statements referring only to women, men, or couples in general or within some normative reference be considered? Should statements about specific people that reflect gender-role behavior be considered?
- How should exceptions, qualifiers, disagreements, and consensus be handled?
- How should the researcher take into account who said what statements and when they were made over the course of the focus group interview?

Other key points for analyzing focus group data are presented in Table 7.11. In addition, observer notes can be used to identify nonverbal behavior that cannot be detected in a transcript.

The extent of analysis of focus group data will depend on the purpose of the focus group and the research questions posed, and whether conclusions can be drawn from

Table 7.11.   Key Dimensions of Analysis
of Focus Group Tape or Transcription[a]

- Changes in question or topic direction
- Group member characteristics
- Language used to describe sexual practices and drug use rituals
- Frequency of responses
- Intensity of responses
- Affective expression; intensity of positive and negative emotion
- Nonverbal body language
- Response themes and subthemes
- Context of responses
- Specificity of response
- Interaction profiles
- Group members' enthusiasm and mood of discussion

[a]From Krueger (1994).

simple analyses (Stewart & Shamdasani, 1990). In addition, availability of resources and time constraints will also drive the comprehensiveness of the analyses.

CONCLUSION

One popular misconception of qualitative data is that it is "soft science" and of little value. As this chapter has illustrated, qualitative data collection and analysis require standards, rigor, and the judgment of trained researchers. Objectivity, auditability, credibility, documentation, and validity are demanded. Alone, qualitative data provide insight into the complexities of living in an environment of HIV risk. In conjunction with quantitative data, they augment the bottom-line analysis provided by "numbers crunching." In other words, qualitative data provide the "flesh to the skeleton" that is quantitative (Anastasi, 1968).

Applying Theory to HIV Prevention Interventions

Theory can inform evaluation research by guiding the development of effective behavior change interventions. This chapter discusses the benefits of incorporating theory with practice and reviews various conceptual frameworks for understanding why individuals engage in health-related behaviors and how health information is diffused. The applicability of particular elements of these theories and models to HIV prevention is also described.

INTEGRATING THEORY AND PRACTICE

Historically, there has been an unnatural disconnection between theory, research, and practice (Hochbaum, Sorenson, & Lorig, 1992). Yet, both practitioners and researchers are accountable for results, whether these are measured in terms of participants' satisfaction with programs or changes in participants' health awareness, behaviors, or quality of life.

Learning and applying theories sometimes can be overwhelming because of the need to review theories from diverse disciplines. Practitioners may have an aversion to developing theory-based interventions because they are constrained by solutions that must be timely, cost-effective, and politically acceptable. These concerns were magnified early in the AIDS epidemic when AIDS researchers and community service providers often had different priorities, perspectives, interests, and agendas (Mantell & DiVittis, 1990; Kelly *et al.*, 1993).

A good theory must answer four questions: (1) What causes the health behavior or condition? (2) How do intervention activities lead to desired health outcomes? (3) How does the interaction among individual, community, and societal factors influence health behavior and conditions? (4) What is the role of the interventionist? (Freudenberg *et al.*, 1995).

Applying theory to practice requires the application and integration of academic skills in a practice environment; adaptation of old theories and models or the development of new ones; and adequate planning time to find a theory or model that fits with the target population, intervention, and evaluation. To facilitate this process, one needs to: (1) identify the target population and the setting in which the intervention will take place; (2) state the behavioral goals and objectives of the intervention; (3) match the models, the target group, and identified goals and objectives; and (4) develop interventions based on the practical constraints of the project. Other issues to be considered are: the

frequency or duration of the target behavior, whether scales or indices to assess constructs exist or have to be created, community-based organizations' (CBOs) accessibility
to experts in various fields for collaboration, and funding for personnel.

THEORY AS A BASIS FOR HIV INTERVENTION

A theory is a systematic group of relationships that can be observed and verified and
that "usually produce particular results under specified conditions" (Hochbaum *et al.*,
1992, p. 296). It explains why an event occurs as it does. These concepts help to explain
what factors might contribute to individual and group behaviors and impact on the
effectiveness of interventions. Theory can help to develop models or generalized descriptions to explain the specific pathways by which an intervention ought to lead to a
desired health-related behavior.

Ineffectiveness of HIV prevention programs has been attributed to both a lack of
theoretical grounding and evaluation (Schaalma, Kok, Braeken, Schoopman, & Deven,
1991). Evaluation of theory-based interventions can enhance practitioners' understanding of why some people adopt and maintain behavior change that eliminates or reduces
their risk of HIV infection while others continue to engage in high-risk activities. Theory
assists health care professionals, individuals, and communities in developing targeted,
cost-effective HIV interventions that can be evaluated and potentially replicated in other
communities and with different populations.

The linkage between health status and behavior contributes to our knowledge about
how to modify HIV-related risks, the biobehavioral basis for and processes of HIV
disease, and the antecedents and consequences of engaging in high-risk activities. Three
approaches to understanding the relationship between health status and behaviors have
been applied to HIV infection: (1) identification of behavioral risk factors and their
relationship to health outcomes; (2) establishment, change, and maintenance of behaviors; and (3) understanding biological mechanisms and their relationship to disease
etiology (Krasnegor, 1990).

A systematic approach is essential for the development of clear behavioral change
goals and intervention objectives and of measures by which to gauge an intervention's
success. Well-established theories emanating from the fields of psychology, sociology,
communications, and education to understand change in behaviors related to smoking,
obesity, and hypertension control have been applied to HIV/AIDS (Lawrence, 1989). In
addition, new HIV-specific models, such as the AIDS risk-reduction model (Catania *et
al.*, 1990b) and the modified AIDS risk-reduction model (Ehrhardt *et al.*, 1992) have been
developed to understand individual determinants of adoption and maintenance of HIV-
related behaviors. Since factors leading to the initiation of a behavior often differ from
those underlying the maintenance of a behavior, theory-based interventions must consider these different stages of behavioral change. Theories developed specifically to
explain community-level HIV risk-related behavioral change have not been established.

Theory-based interventions enable the health professional to pinpoint specific
program components that might be effective or noneffective for specific populations. For
example, most HIV-related intervention studies have shown knowledge to be important

but not sufficient in health behavior change. This gap between cognition and behavior challenges program planners to find a way to translate increased knowledge into preventive actions.

THEORIES AND MODELS OF HEALTH-RELATED BEHAVIOR

In this section, we review 13 theories and models that have been applied to HIV-related behavior with varying degrees of success. They are: (1) the health belief model (Rosenstock, 1974; Maiman & Becker, 1974); (2) social learning/social–cognitive theory (Bandura, 1977a,b, 1986); (3) the theory of reasoned action (Fishbein & Ajzen, 1975); (4) protection motivation theory (Rogers, 1975); (5) relapse prevention theory (Marlatt & Gordon, 1985); (6) transtheoretical or stages of behavioral change model (Prochaska & DiClemente, 1983, 1986); (7) AIDS risk reduction model (Catania *et al.*, 1990b); (8) modified AIDS risk reduction model (Ehrhardt *et al.*, 1992); (9) diffusion of innovation model (Rogers, 1983); (10) social action theory (Ewart, 1991, 1995); (11) organizational stage theory (Kaluzny & Hernandez, 1988); (12) organizational development theory (Tichy & Beckhard, 1982; Brown & Covey, 1987); and (13) the PRECEDE–PROCEED model (Green & Kreuter, 1991). The discussion of theories and models is categorized according to whether they are individual- or community-level type. Numbers 1 to 5 are cognitive individual-level models and theories 6 to 8 are stage individual models and theories. The last five 9 through 13, are community-level, or macro, models and theories.

The development, components, application to HIV, and strengths and weaknesses of each theory/model are presented. Limitations of these models and recommendations for future application of models to interventions are addressed.

Individual-Level Cognitive Models and Theories

The Health Belief Model

The health belief model (HBM) is the most commonly used model to predict and explain individual health behaviors (Hochbaum, 1958; Rosenstock, 1966, 1974; Becker & Maiman, 1975; Janz & Becker, 1984). This cognitive learning theory focuses on health-related perceptions and motivations and applies a cost-benefit perspective to explain preventive health behaviors. The HBM states that health behavior is a function of the individual's perception and the interaction of: (1) threat (susceptibility to and severity of illness); (2) outcome expectations (preventive benefits weighed against perceived barriers to behavioral change, such as practical and emotional costs of the prescribed behavior); and (3) cue to action in the form of internal (e.g., physical symptoms) or external (e.g., social experience) stimuli (Rosenstock, 1974; Maiman & Becker, 1974) (see Fig. 8.1).

Lewin's (1951) value-expectancy theory explains behavior as the resulting sum of positive and negative forces on the individual. Based on this theory, the HBM was initially developed by social scientists working for the US Public Health Service in the

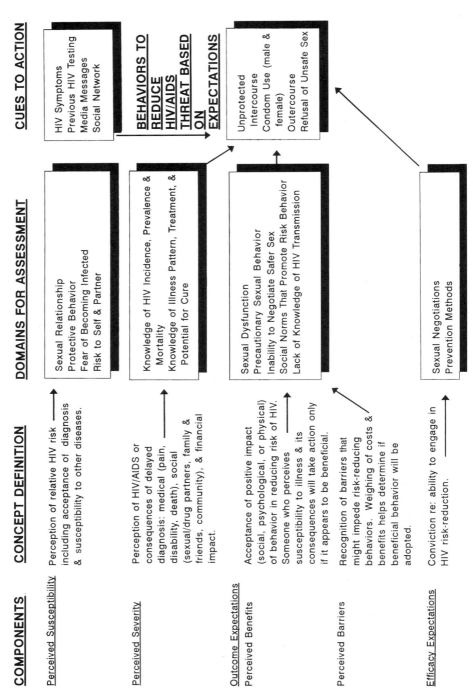

Figure 8.1. Health belief model applied to HIV sexual risk-reduction behavior.

1950s to explain why persons did not participate in free mobile X-ray screening for tuberculosis. Subsequently, the model was applied to explain preventive behaviors, such as influenza immunization (Rosenstock, 1966), children's dietary behavior (Becker, Maiman, Kirscht, Haefner, & Drachman, 1977), and breast self-examination (Hallal, 1982). Janz and Becker's (1984) comprehensive literature review of prospective and retrospective research studies on the HBM from 1974 through 1984 showed that perceived barriers was the most predictive component, while perceived severity was the least predictive component across a range of health-related behaviors.

The concept of self-efficacy, the "conviction that one can successfully execute the behavior required to produce the outcomes" (Bandura, 1977a,b, 1986), was integrated into the model in the 1980s (Maiman & Becker, 1974; Rosenstock, Strecher, & Becker, 1988). The updated HBM assumes that individuals must feel the need to change (perceived susceptibility and severity) and believe that the change will be advantageous, and that they are competent to make the change.

Applications to AIDS. The utility of the various components of the HBM in predicting HIV risk-reduction behavior among gay men, injection drug users (Becker & Joseph, 1988), and adolescents has been inconsistent (Petosa & Jackson, 1991). Some studies have shown contradictory effects of perceived susceptibility and health behavior (greater perceived risk associated with greater likelihood of adopting the health behavior, e.g., Aspinwall, Kemeny, Taylor, Schneider, & Dudley, 1991; Hingson, Strunin, Berlin, & Heeren, 1990; Basen-Enquist & Parcel, 1992; versus no relationship between the two variables, e.g., Brown, DiClemente, & Reynolds, 1991; Walter *et al.*, 1992; Montgomery *et al.*, 1989; Huang, Watters, & Case, 1989). Similarly, the effects of perceived severity of HIV/AIDS on HIV prevention behavior have been inconsistent [high perceived severity was associated with the adoption of HIV prevention behavior (e.g., Montgomery *et al.*, 1989) versus no relationship between the two variables (e.g., Catania *et al.*, 1990b)]. With respect to adoption of needle-use risk-reduction behaviors, at least three studies of injection drug users found that avoidance of AIDS (an indirect measure of susceptibility) was a significant factor (Des Jarlais, Friedman, & Hopkins, 1985; Friedman, 1987; Ginzburg *et al.*, 1986).

Early in the epidemic, an inverse association was reported between having seen a debilitated person with AIDS and likelihood of high-risk sexual practices in gay men (McKusick, Horstman, & Coates, 1985; Bye, 1987); this was interpreted as evidence of the role of perceived susceptibility and severity. Studies that report no relationship between severity and HIV-related behaviors may be, in part, a function of the way severity has been measured. Measures of severity have focused on death and anxiety, but few have looked at quality of life issues, such as rejection and isolation (Rosenstock, Strecher, & Becker, 1994). Gender may also determine whether components of the HBM are significant.

Even the updated HBM has several shortcomings: (1) it does not address the influence of culture, class, economics, environment, and life experience in shaping health behaviors; (2) it fails to consider the role of both habit and social network influence in health behavior decisions; and (3) it does not provide recommendations for ways to persuade persons to change their behaviors (Siegel, Grodsky, & Herman, 1986).

In addition, the HBM does not examine the interaction between multiple risk behaviors (i.e., sex and drugs) and its impact on HIV risk and precautionary behaviors, the dyadic nature of sexual behavior, and maintenance of behavioral change over time. An additional limitation unique to adolescents is that the HBM constructs are insensitive to maturational issues (Brown *et al.*, 1991).

Social Learning Theory

Social learning/social–cognitive theory (SLT) assumes that behavior and environment are best studied as reciprocal systems that interact continuously. Environment shapes, supports, and constrains behavior, while people create their surroundings. Key concepts of the theory are reciprocal determinism (interaction among a person, his or her behavior, and the environment in which the behavior takes place), behavioral capability, expectations, self-efficacy, observational learning, and reinforcement (Glanz, Lewis, & Rimer, 1990). Individual learning and behavior are achieved by (1) direct experience; (2) indirect experience (from observation or modeling); (3) storing and processing complex information that enables one to anticipate the consequences of actions; (4) skills enhancement (rehearsal and feedback); and (5) social support (reinforcement, especially from one's peers) (Bandura, 1990).

Self-efficacy, one aspect of the social learning framework, has been an important mediating factor between health attitudes and beliefs and behavioral change (Bandura, 1977b; O'Leary, 1985; DiClemente, Prochaska, & Gilbertini, 1985). To implement protective health behaviors, one needs to have not only compelling reasons, but knowledge, resources, social supports, and skills. Self-efficacy is behavior-specific and does not necessarily extend to all health behavior situations (Bandura, 1977a,b). Factors such as previous observations and reinforcement experience, coupled with perceptions of the environment, may impact positively or negatively on one's self-efficacy. The likelihood of adopting a health behavior is a function of an interaction of expectations about the outcomes that will result from the behavior and expectations about one's ability to carry out the behavior (Green & Kreuter, 1991).

Sources of self-efficacy include: (1) performance attainment; (2) vicarious learning; (3) social persuasion; and (4) physiological information. Change strategies derived from self-efficacy theory include modeling, incremental goal-setting, behavior contracting, feedback, self-monitoring, verbal persuasion, and encouragement (Green & Kreuter, 1991). Modeling has been found to be an important component in behavior change in studies of new mothers' ability to parent (Unger & Wandersman, 1985) and cardiovascular patients' ability to protect themselves from heart disease (Levy, 1983).

This theory proposes that behavior is determined by expectations and incentives. Performance attainment and self-confidence can be enhanced by dividing a target behavior into manageable steps with repetitive tasks that are monitored and reinforced. Increased familiarity and comfort based on successfully completing incremental tasks encourage initiation and continuation of behaviors that promote change. By mastering consecutive steps building toward a desired behavior, even if a person fails at one step or lapses along the way, he or she can appraise why goals were not met and can reinitiate the process.

The theory is a self-control approach that posits that an individual can learn cognitive–behavioral skills to cope competently with conditions that may trigger relapse (Marlatt & Gordon, 1985). Behavioral coping skills training and cognitive restructuring techniques are the foundation of interventions geared to changing patterns of sexual expression and drug use. Problem-solving exercises help strengthen the individual's ability to define problem situations and weigh the benefits and costs of implementing alternative strategies. Self-management consists of developing contingency plans and contracts and action plans for rejecting or avoiding high-risk behaviors. Role plays are used to help rehearse response alternatives to stressful situations that might be likely to trigger relapse. Buddy systems may be used to reinforce peer support.

The goal of BRP is to prevent a single lapse or complete relapse as well as to promote a healthy lifestyle. Relapse is usually related to a high-risk situation, such as (1) negative emotional state, (2) interpersonal conflict, or (3) social pressure (direct or indirect) to return to the old behavior. After relapse, decreased perception of risk is an important factor in continuing the relapse behavior (Gibbons *et al.*, 1991). This would seem to suggest that intervention needs to focus on maintaining or increasing perceptions of risk.

Stage Models

Transtheoretical or Stages of Change Model

A model of intentional stages of behavioral change was developed to understand addictive disorders, such as smoking and drug and alcohol addiction (DiClemente, 1986; DiClemente & Prochaska, 1982). The transtheoretical model (TM), unlike the previously described models, suggests that individuals pass through stages in considering health-related behaviors, and that the determinants of each of these stages differ. It is a three-dimensional model that addresses: (1) stages (when changes occur), (2) processes (how individuals make changes), and (3) levels of behavioral change (what people change), from initial adoption to maintenance.

During the past 14 years, the number of stages of the model has been altered from five to four back to five. Currently, the concept of preparation for change has been added to the model. The current stages of change in Prochaska and DiClemente's (1992) model applied to HIV prevention are described below and also shown in Fig. 8.3.

Individuals do not necessarily go through the stages of change in a linear fashion, and may be in more than one stage of change simultaneously. The model also posits that the relative importance of change varies within each stage:

1. Stage 1: Precontemplation. There may be a wish to change but there is no clear intent to change behavior in the near future (approximately 6 months). Individuals are not ready for self-evaluation and are typically resistant to changing their behavior. They are unaware of their risk and choose to deny that something deleterious might happen to them as a result of their health behavior.
2. Stage 2: Contemplation. The individual may be aware of a problem and be seriously thinking about how to overcome it. Intentions to change their behavior are formed, but there is no commitment to behavior change. A person can be

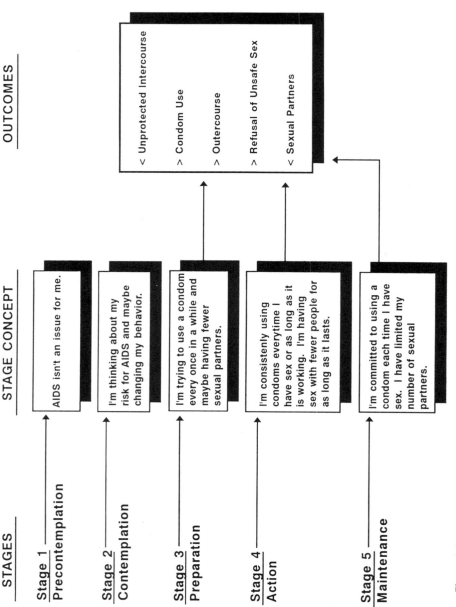

Figure 8.3. The transtheoretical model (TM) of change applied to HIV prevention. (Adapted from Prochaska & DiClemente, 1992.)

in this stage for extended periods of time. Consciousness-raising processes, such as observation, confrontation, and interpretation, are widely used.

3. Stage 3: Preparation. Initial steps toward reducing the frequency of the behavior have begun; some change may be initiated. The individual seriously commits to changing the behavior within a month.

4. Stage 4: Action. The individual modifies a specific or a group of behaviors for a predetermined amount of time. This phase can be divided into early-action (0–3 months) and late action (4–6 months). Self-liberation, counterconditioning, and conditional stimuli are emphasized, and though people have begun to change their behavior, such change may be inconsistent.

5. Stage 5: Maintenance. Once a behavior has been successfully changed for 6 months, the individual is in the final phase of behavior change. The person is able to incorporate the behavior change continually into his or her daily life. Successful maintenance is often challenged by interpersonal and environmental factors that encourage the old behavior.

Relapse is most often found in the action stage, but it does not entail a permanent return to the negative behavior. The majority of people relapse and return to the precontemplation or contemplation stage before moving on (Prochaska, Redding, Harlow, Rossi, & Velicer, 1994). Relapse can also occur in the maintenance stage. Each stage builds on the strengths of the previous stage of change. Change at one level is likely to produce change at another level. The model is an improvement over a one-step model of behavioral change because of its recognition that change may be gradual, dynamic, and continual. The TM is focused on interpersonal behavioral change and fails to consider structural influences on behavior.

AIDS-specific heuristic frameworks incorporating stages of behavioral change, such as the AIDS risk-reduction model (Catania *et al.*, 1990b) and the modified AIDS risk-reduction (Ehrhardt *et al.*, 1992), have been developed to explain the initial adoption of a behavioral change and most importantly how such change is maintained over time.

Theoretical models of HIV prevention have focused heavily on cognitive variables, often not taking into account the mediating role of social influence processes and contextual factors, i.e., social norms, social networks, the media, community and organizational participation, gender roles, culture, and power, in bringing about changes in sexual and drug-related behaviors. The AIDS risk-reduction and modified AIDS risk-reduction models address these issues.

AIDS Risk-Reduction Model

The AIDS risk-reduction model (ARRM) (Catania *et al.*, 1990b) integrates elements of the HBM (Becker, 1974; Janz & Becker, 1984), SLT (Bandura, 1977a,b, 1989), TRA (Fishbein & Ajzen, 1975), and TM (Prochaska & DiClemente, 1986) to explain AIDS preventive actions. It acknowledges behavior change as a multistep process with different psychological and social determinants for each stage.

Though originally designed to predict sexual risk reduction, the ARRM can be modified to predict drug-related risk reduction. Important factors are: (1) knowledge of risk levels of sexual activities and ways to make low-risk behaviors more satisfying; (2) perceptions of HIV risk susceptibility; (3) perceived cost–benefits of reduced high-risk behavior; (4) self-efficacy beliefs; (5) emotional states; and (6) social factors, including group norms, social support, help-seeking, and communication skills (Catania *et al.*, 1990b). In addition to factors such as peer norms, knowledge, and self-efficacy, the ARRM emphasizes the roles of help-seeking behavior and aversive emotions in the enactment of safer sex practices.

The model views behavior change proceeding in three stages, as described below:

1. Labeling of high-risk behavior. Individuals become knowledgeable about HIV transmission and acknowledge their HIV risk behaviors. Knowledge, perceived susceptibility, social networks, and norms are important determinants of this stage.
2. Commitment to changing high-risk behavior. Individuals make decisions based on the costs and benefits, which include the perceived effectiveness of reducing HIV risk behaviors (response efficacy) and the pleasure associated with them. Persons learn effective ways to reduce their risk and dedicate themselves to perform risk-reducing behaviors. Thus, both response efficacy and self-efficacy are key elements in this stage.
3. Enactment of risk-reduction behavior. Individuals seek ways to commence action toward changing their high-risk behaviors. Communication skills and peer support play important roles. Each prevention strategy must be matched to the developmental stage of each target audience.

Movement from one stage to another is predicated upon achieving the goals and objectives of the prior stage. Emotions, alcohol and drug use, and environmental clues impact behavior motivation over time. It is imperative to understand the different conditions that influence the outcomes of the various stages of the change process. This informs intervention strategies that facilitate movement toward change for people at different stages in the process. Although the ARRM has been applied to gay men, it is also applicable to diverse populations such as bisexuals, heterosexuals, teens, and communities of color (Kegeles, Coates, Christopher, & Lazarus, 1989).

As the role of sexuality to personal identity and its contribution to relationships had not been recognized by other behavior models, Ehrhardt and colleagues (1992) modified the ARRM to be specific to explaining sexual behavior change, as described below.

Modified AIDS Risk-Reduction Model

The modified AIDS risk-reduction model (M-ARRM) is another model of stages of behavioral change that is an integral part of the project "Sexual Risk Behavior and Behavior Change in Heterosexual Women and Men" at the HIV Center for Clinical and Behavioral Studies, New York State Psychiatric Institute (Ehrhardt *et al.*, 1992). The M-ARRM includes elements of the ARRM (Catania *et al.*, 1990b) and adds new components based on extensive research with heterosexual women and men, as shown in Fig. 8.4. The model posits that there are different determinants for each stage of behavior change because of the complexity of sexual risk behavior.

In the M-ARRM, the labeling stage of the ARRM has been renamed the *suscep-*

issues, the value orientations of influential persons and groups, the environment within an organization or community, and the constraints and sources of resistance to change.

Organizational Development Theory

Organizational development theory (Tichy & Beckhard, 1982) addresses some of the limitations of organizational stage theory. It seeks to identify problems that are barriers to the organization's healthy functioning, rather than to initiate specific behaviors. Intervention is directed toward changing organizational processes and structures and workers' behavior and roles so as to improve organizational effectiveness (Brown & Covey, 1987). Quality of life issues and human relationships are often the targets of problem diagnosis, action planning (development of interventions to address problems identified), interventions (development of team-building strategies, process consultation), and evaluation (assessment of planned change). In addition, the roles of environmental factors and an organization's cultural values, ideologies, and social norms in effecting organizational change are addressed.

Both organizational stage and organization development theories can guide the development of specific intervention strategies tailored to a community's stage of readiness and can identify appropriate community leaders, health care providers, and groups that would be most likely to promote community-wide HIV behavioral change. To date, we are unaware of any community-level HIV preventive interventions built on an organizational theory framework.

PRECEDE–PROCEED Model

A meta-paradigm that combines many of the previously mentioned concepts is the PRECEDE–PROCEED model (PPM) developed by Green and Kreuter (1991), shown in Fig. 8.6. This comprehensive planning model provides a framework for assessing a community's needs. It identifies factors that contribute to health problems that must be changed to initiate and sustain the process of behavioral and environmental change, analyzes policies and resources that can facilitate or hinder development of health promotion programs, and identifies strategies for implementation and evaluation of interventions. Although it may seem that the model begins at the end (outcomes) rather than the beginning (inputs), for planning needs it is essential to identify potential determinants of an outcome before an intervention is designed. The nine phases of PPM are:

1. Phase 1. Social diagnosis: Quality-of-life issues, which are the subjective problems and priorities of the individual or the community, are addressed. A practical way to distinguish characteristics of one's life is to study social and health states.
2. Phase 2. Epidemiological diagnosis: This phase addresses the health of the individual or the community by looking at vital indicators such as morbidity, mortality, disability, and fertility. The health problems are prioritized according to the magnitude and severity, its risk to special subsets of the population, its economic impact, the ability to reduce the burden of disease, and whether it is being addressed by other organizations.

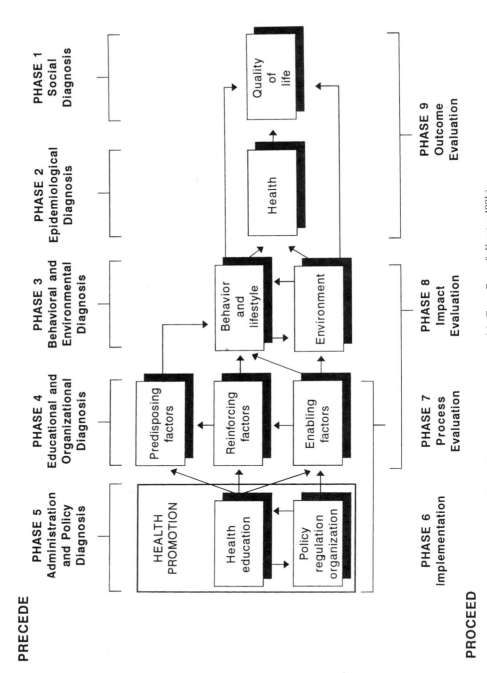

Figure 8.6. PRECEDE–PROCEED model. (From Green & Kreuter, 1991.)

3. Phase 3. Behavioral and environmental diagnosis: Behavioral and environmental indicators of health, such as risk factors, are identified and ranked. It is important to understand the environmental context and its impact on personal behavior.

4. Phase 4. Educational and organizational diagnosis: This stage delineates the predisposing (knowledge, attitudes, beliefs, values), enabling (availability and access to health and social services, supportive governmental policies, and health-related skills), and reinforcing (supportive family, colleagues, friends, communities, and health and social service providers) factors that facilitate or hinder the motivation for change and its maintenance. These factors which affect the desired behavior change and the environment are ranked.

5. Phase 5. Administrative and policy diagnosis: This stage involves a critical evaluation of the capabilities and resources available and barriers to implementing a program. It includes budget, personnel, policies, and time constraints of the service providers and organizations as well as the linkages with the community.

6. Phase 6. Implementation: The plan is converted into health education intervention, policy, organization, and regulation.

7. Phase 7. Process evaluation: This occurs because early identification of problems in a feedback loop helps the educator to adjust program content, teaching styles, and presentations and materials.

8. Phase 8. Impact evaluation: This type of evaluation directly assesses the effect of the educational intervention, which includes changes in predisposing, enabling, and reinforcing factors of behavioral/environmental changes.

9. Phase 9. Outcome evaluation: The effect of the intervention on long-term changes in quality of life, social indicators, disability, and morbidity or mortality rates is assessed.

Social and epidemiological diagnoses are often used as the basis for a community needs assessment (see Chapter 4). Additionally, many health care providers are interested in educational and organizational diagnoses. Predisposing factors are established personal or community traits that impact on behavior change, including knowledge, attitudes, beliefs, values, and perceptions. Enabling factors are created by societal factors and environmental factors. To support behavior changes successfully, certain services and supports, such as availability and accessibility of health personnel and resources, established policies, and laws that show commitment to health and personal ability to perform health skills, must exist. Reinforcing factors help maintain behavior change. They include positive reinforcement, such as praise and reassurance and continuing rewards, as well as social support that helps one initiate and maintain behavior change. Reinforcers include family members, friends, peers, employers, teachers, co-workers, health personnel, community leaders, and policymakers.

When these specific factors are understood, objectives, criteria, and evaluation mechanisms can be focused on the specific population to be educated (Green & Kreuter, 1991). This model has been validated and applied successfully in a variety of areas, including adoption of seatbelts (Gielen & Radius, 1984), planning for maternal and child health programs (Green et al., 1978), and nutrition and cancer education (Light & Contento, 1989). By focusing on behavioral and health outcomes, it is useful for the development of HIV preventive interventions. The PROCEED component of the model helps to develop and initiate evaluation and policy development.

Application to AIDS.   Freudenberg (1989) used the PRECEDE model to develop objectives to decrease the incidence of new HIV infections among women enrolled in a drug treatment program. Intervention objectives were to discuss alternative stress-reduction techniques, identify sources of peer and social support for continued drug-free behavior, and inform women about perinatal HIV transmission. These objectives were translated into intervention activities that included support groups, peer educator training, demonstrations of cleaning drug-related paraphernalia, and small-group discussions on AIDS and reproductive decisions. Three indicators of intervention impact were identified: use of condoms, cessation of drug use, and, for women who continued to inject drugs, sterilization of needles or participation in a needle-exchange programs. The PROCEED phase focuses on implementing and evaluating the program.

The PRECEDE component of the model in relation to AIDS is shown in Fig. 8.7.

DIRECTIONS FOR FUTURE THEORY DEVELOPMENT

Although some existing theories and models have been applied to AIDS prevention, they have had limited success in explaining HIV-related behaviors. A theory or model is a guide to explaining behavioral change. It is not written in stone, and hence should not limit the program developer. He or she can modify, combine, and adapt theories to explain behavioral change. Each theory or model may have useful features, but a combination will be more successful in guiding interventions (Kirscht & Joseph, 1989; Ewart, 1995).

At a 1991 National Institute of Mental Health-sponsored Theorist Workshop (Fishbein *et al.*, 1991) attended by creators of theories and models, including Fishbein, Bandura, Becker and Middlestadt, eight variables that account for variations in HIV-related behavior were identified: (1) intentions; (2) environmental constraints; (3) ability (skills); (4) anticipated outcomes (or attitudes); (5) norms; (6) self-standards; (7) emotions; and (8) self-efficacy. There was no consensus, however, as to the causal relations among these variables. However, intentions were generally seen as being the most proximal to behavior and the other variables were seen as influencing the formation and strength of intentions and/or as influencing the likelihood that one will act upon his or her intentions.

To understand determinants of HIV-related behavioral change, variables in addition to the eight described above must be addressed and focus should be on the community as well as the individual. The specific variables we believe must be addressed are cultural background and orientation, socioeconomic status, gender roles, and power in relationships. There is little understanding of how specific social and economic situations enhance or reduce risk behavior and how the complex social behavior of partners and social network members shape and influence HIV-related prevention and risk-reduction behaviors. This more inclusive approach will become the building blocks for successful theory-based interventions.

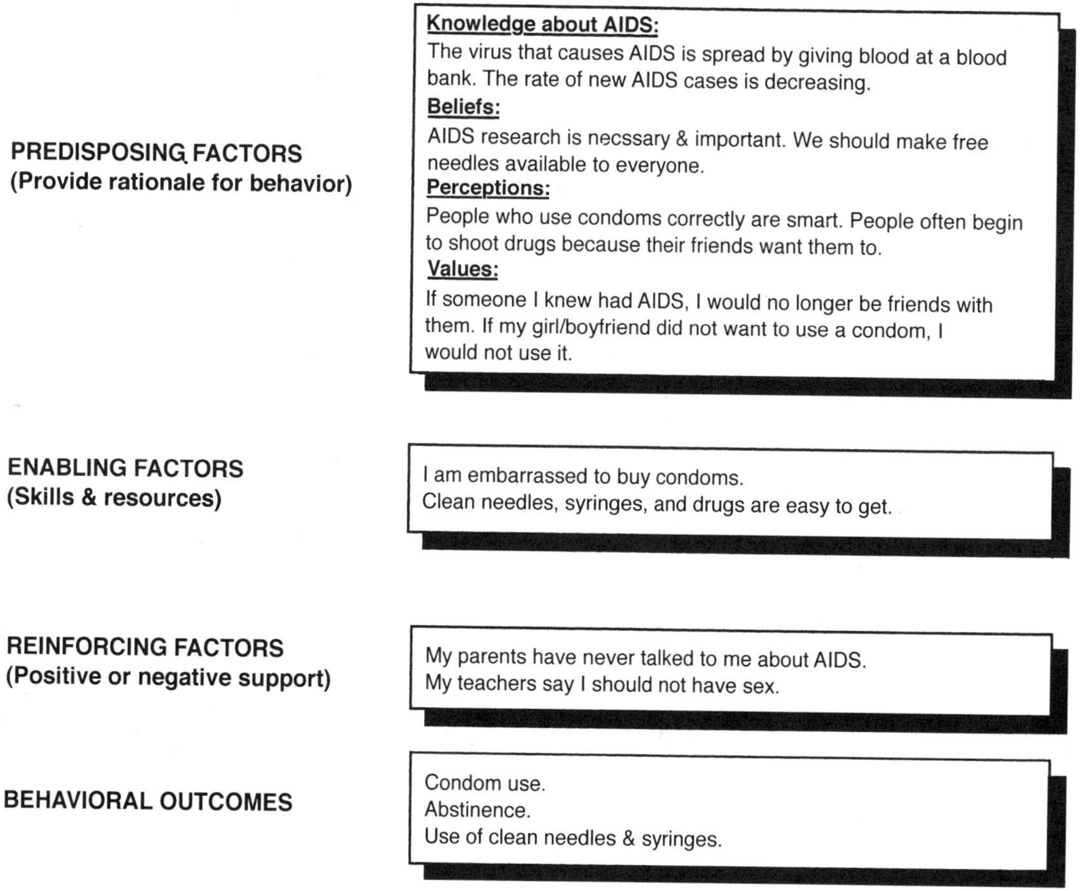

**PREDISPOSING FACTORS
(Provide rationale for behavior)**

Knowledge about AIDS:
The virus that causes AIDS is spread by giving blood at a blood bank. The rate of new AIDS cases is decreasing.
Beliefs:
AIDS research is necssary & important. We should make free needles available to everyone.
Perceptions:
People who use condoms correctly are smart. People often begin to shoot drugs because their friends want them to.
Values:
If someone I knew had AIDS, I would no longer be friends with them. If my girl/boyfriend did not want to use a condom, I would not use it.

**ENABLING FACTORS
(Skills & resources)**

I am embarrassed to buy condoms.
Clean needles, syringes, and drugs are easy to get.

**REINFORCING FACTORS
(Positive or negative support)**

My parents have never talked to me about AIDS.
My teachers say I should not have sex.

BEHAVIORAL OUTCOMES

Condom use.
Abstinence.
Use of clean needles & syringes.

Figure 8.7. PRECEDE model applied to junior high school students HIV-related knowledge, attitudes, beliefs, and behaviors. (Adapted from Alteneder, Price, Telljohann, Didion, & Locher, 1992.)

CONCLUSION

Basing preventive interventions on a theory or model goes beyond an academic exercise. Its purpose is to understand better the mechanisms of health behavioral change and maintenance. This enables the program developer to design an intervention that will capitalize on the theorized determinants of behavior change. A program grounded in a theory enables the evaluator to focus the evaluation in terms of identifying indicators of change for the impact and outcome evaluation. Further, the evaluation of the program can test the fit of the model to the data. From there, the next generation of models is formulated, improving the next generation of interventions.

Evaluating Individual-Level and Community-Level Interventions

PLANNING FOR THE EVALUATION OF AN INTERVENTION

Evaluating an intervention is more than coming up with a scientifically sound design, data collection strategies, and measures. Before implementing an intervention, a number of decisions have to be thought through carefully. All components of the intervention have to fit and be closely linked. The evaluation protocol for the intervention also has to be practical. Whatever intervention is chosen is dependent on the behavior you want to promote, the audience to be reached, and the acceptability of the intervention to the population.

Failure to address these issues can lead to an ineffective intervention. When an evaluator is involved in the initial planning and design of an intervention, he or she is provided with a comprehensive overview. A key challenge in the planning and decision-making processes is to ensure that all the parts work and are interdependent. Clearly, getting in on the ground floor helps. Below, we review key phases to be considered in the planning and design process of interventions that will facilitate evaluation (adapted from S. Miller, 1995).

- Define the problem. Pinpoint the behavioral deficits, and the behaviors to be learned that will lead to the ideal behavior; identify unmet needs, cultural values, and appropriate modes for intervention.
- Select and analyze the target groups. The primary target group is population-specific, such as homeless women living on the streets, gay and bisexual men of color, adolescents, and family-planning service providers. At another level, the target group represents the larger unit, e.g., partners, peers, families, organizations, and communities for whom the intervention will be effective. Sometimes interventions should also be directed to a secondary target group known to influence the primary target group. This would include peers, sex workers, opinion leaders, sexual partners, family members, and public figures. These sources of influence may facilitate or impede behavioral change. Intervention may be directed to this group only, rather than the primary target group.
- Determine needed resources and costs. What are the costs associated with implementing the intervention? This includes consideration of personnel, space, equipment, and financial incentives for participation (e.g., transportation, child care, food).
- Establish the research and intervention structures. This includes choosing a

205

theoretical framework, laying the groundwork for forming a research team, and considering study design and intervention issues. In particular, decisions need to be made about how to translate intervention objectives into activities and measurable behavioral objectives. As discussed in Chapter 8, the theoretical framework guides the intervention.

- Design research and intervention protocols. This includes the goals, objectives, methods, measures, and assessment methods:

    1. Barriers to intervention. Identifying the potential barriers to intervention is perhaps one of the most important tasks to be tackled. Barriers might be related to race/ethnicity, gender, class, safety, ease of travel, legal, employment constraints, literacy level, organizational policies, and vested interests. Anticipating these obstacles and deriving solutions can help ensure that appropriate decisions are made with respect to selection of the setting, level of intimacy, frequency, duration of contact with participants, and recruitment strategies.

    2. Linking intervention with outcomes. There should always be a direct correspondence among the intervention objectives, measures, and outcomes. For example, if the intervention is expected to increase knowledge, change social norms, increase motivation for HIV risk reduction, and increase protected sex, the outcomes should be assessed accordingly.

    3. Desired level of intimacy. The intervention can be conducted face-to-face with individuals or groups, by mail, by telephone, video, or mass media. Based on knowledge of the target population, the level of intimacy is determined.

    4. Setting. Decisions about where the intervention should take place must be made. Potential settings include health clinics, hospitals, shelters, drug treatment centers, on the streets, community-based organizations, housing projects, and single-room occupancy hotels. The setting should maximize participation by providing access, comfort, and safety.

    5. Comprehensiveness. Does the intervention stand on its own or is it part of a larger intervention strategy? For example, is a school-based sex education program for adolescents being implemented independently or as part of a larger health promotion curriculum?

    6. Intensity. Frequency of contact with participants, length of each contact, and interval between contacts are indicators of the intensity of the intervention. In determining appropriate intensity, the nature of the target group must be considered. For example, it may be unrealistic to expect that service providers can attend daily sessions of a counseling workshop delivered over a 2-week period.

    7. Intervention modes. Examples of intervention modes include lecture/discussion, videos and slide shows, one-to-one counseling, problem-solving skills training groups, support groups, peer outreach, needle exchange, and mass media (e.g., public service announcements).

    8. Recruitment strategies. Are the recruitment process and intervention compatible and mutually supportive?

- Pretest the intervention, materials, and assessment schedule. Prior to implementing the intervention, a test run should be conducted to assess the effectiveness of the recruitment strategies, intervention logistics, procedures, format and flow, appeal and cultural sensitivity, and clarity of materials.
- Monitor the intervention. Strategies for monitoring the intervention need to be in place. Decisions regarding the use of questionnaires, checklists, or participant observation need to be made before the onset of the intervention in order for the evaluator to assess the formative and summative outcomes.
- Evaluate findings. The development of an analysis plan prior to data collection will enable the evaluator to answer research questions in a timely and unbiased manner.
- Modify the intervention. Specific feedback loops for feeding formative evaluation results into program modification need to be identified and in place prior to implementation. There should be specific times (e.g., between intervention cycles) when modifications can be made without jeopardizing the intervention. It is important to route information to not only the program designers, but to the steering committees, key leaders, and community representatives.
- Implement the intervention in multiple settings. Testing the generalizablity of the intervention across setting attests to the utility of the intervention. Can the intervention be replicated in other settings? How will others view the utility of the intervention and decide to implement it? What is the plan for disseminating intervention findings?

The aforementioned points illustrate and reinforce the necessary partnership between the community, program developer, and the evaluator. Before we review the evaluation of specific intervention strategies, we will discuss the use of social marketing and incentives in targeting a sample and retaining them in the intervention.

SOCIAL MARKETING

Social marketing, widely used by market researchers to increase the acceptability of an idea, innovation, product, or social behavior (Kotler & Zaltman, 1971), is being increasingly used as a strategy in the planning process, design, and dissemination of HIV prevention programs. Its major focus is on the user of the product and how to maximize the perceived benefits of the product. Market research strategies help identify segments, product distribution, outlets/channels, features, product price (i.e., economic, social, and psychological barriers), and promotion strategies to guide systematic decision-making. These in turn are used in the design of credible messages and the selection of information channels for targeted advertising campaigns to best reach specific consumer populations. The intent is to assess the benefits and costs that influence a persons's willingness to change behavior. Both quantitative and qualitative methods, including focus groups, indepth interviews, and surveys, can be employed to understand user behavior.

To identify population-specific information about potential consumers of the product and sources, messages, and channels for reaching a population engaged in high risk behaviors, audiences are segmented into groups with shared characteristics (Slater & Flora, 1991). For example, prior to initiating an AIDS education program for residents in drug treatment, program staff held a series of focus groups to identify educational materials that would be relevant and sensitive to the needs of the audience (Mantell *et al.*, 1989a). Evaluating audience reactions to HIV prevention messages can tell educators and researchers how to aim messages better and which channels of communication should be used so that the program will be well received by the intended audience.

In Example 9.1, social marketing was used to explore the potential for informal community networks to serve as a channel for disseminating HIV prevention information. Similar strategies could be employed in the United States, in venues that people frequent during the course of their daily activities such as light assembly and garment factories, *bodegas* (grocery stores), *botanicas* (natural medicine stores) and pharmacies, and housing projects.

Once the appropriate prevention messages have been determined, social marketing can be used to promote specific components of a prevention campaign, e.g., how to increase the availability and use of condoms and other contraceptive methods and identify appropriate channels. The relative advantage perceived by a population and the barriers to buying and using condoms can be identified. Through this type of research, the evaluator may also learn how condoms should be packaged to appeal to women and what norms will motivate them to influence their partners to use condoms. Research findings might also indicate that condoms can be promoted effectively through television and radio advertising, billboards, subway and bus posters, pharmacy display, and with attractive packaging techniques. They might also show that less expensive channels,

---

Example 9.1.   Social Marketing in South Africa

Evaluation Strategy

An exploratory survey of 88 shopkeepers who sold packaged food and daily supplies in the black South African township of Khayelitsha was conducted to determine their potential for disseminating HIV prevention information and condoms. All shops up to three buildings deep along the main road of two different locales were surveyed. Structured personal interviews were conducted in both English and Xhosa. The degree to which shopkeepers served as opinion leaders and influenced customers about health care products and the types of information exchanged was assessed.

Results

Over three quarters of the shopkeepers reported that their customers sought advice on health products from them. All consented to distribute AIDS education pamphlets and posters in their stores; nearly 90% indicated that they would be willing to sell condoms and would continue to do so if their customers purchased them. About one third of the shopkeepers belonged to a business network. Based on survey results, the researchers concluded that shopkeepers were respected opinion leaders in the community, and thus represented an untapped, influential source for condom distribution.

(SOURCE: Marks & Downes, 1991.)

which utilize neighborhood venues such as beauty parlors and laundromats, would be useful.

One example of an innovative social marketing campaign was the joint initiative between a drinks company (Société Centrafricaine des Boissons) and a US-based nonprofit organization (PSI) in which four-packs of condoms were exchanged for five bottle tops (World Health Organization Global Programme on AIDS, 1993). As part of the promotional campaign, music was played in the markets and bars, promotional items were given away, and informational sessions and condom demonstrations were provided.

With the chronic nature of HIV, social marketing can increasingly play a role in disease prevention strategies. Unfortunately, there is a dearth of systematic attempts to evaluate the effectiveness of social marketing interventions in the area of AIDS. This is especially true in relation to the influence of socially advertised prevention messages on sexual behavior (Wyld & Hallock, 1989). Social marketing is one of many strategies that can be mobilized in the dissemination and evaluation of prevention campaigns. Other broader intervention strategies that may be equally or more effective include changing peer and community social norms, advocating health-promoting public policy and legislation, building community infrastructures and coalitions, developing alliances with media officials, and supporting grass roots community health participation (Ling, Franklin, Lindsteadt, & Gearon, 1992).

ENROLLMENT AND RETENTION: USING INCENTIVES TO RECRUIT AND RETAIN SUBJECTS IN INTERVENTIONS

Providing participants with incentives to enroll in research studies is a controversial issue. Below, we outline some of the major arguments for using incentives as well as concerns about their use. Techniques used to recruit subjects are of interest to the evaluator because they can affect study design, validity, and program success. Recruitment efforts in several studies of homosexual and bisexual men (e.g., the Pitt Men's Study in Pittsburgh and several studies in the Gay Men's Health Crisis Research Program) have resulted in skewed samples of middle-class, white, gay men who made significant changes in their sexual behaviors prior to program participation. Thus, incentives to draw and retain men of color, as well as men who have sex with men but do not identify themselves as gay or bisexual in behavioral research programs are needed. Monetary incentives may be more useful for stimulating initial participation in a study and for programs targeting acquisition rather than maintenance of knowledge and skills (Winett, King, & Altman, 1989).

Advantages

Researchers often need to offer incentives to encourage subjects' initial participation or retention in a study over time. Such "aggressive" recruitment strategies aim to serve as positive reinforcement to engage and motivate participants' interest in the program. For purposes of evaluation, the effects of providing incentives on response and return rates should be monitored.

Careful consideration should be given, however, to what the incentive is, its significance to HIV prevention, cultural appropriateness to the target population, and when it is distributed to program participants (e.g., before or after the intervention). Conducting focus groups with both staff and target group members is one way to determine appropriate incentives. Another issue relates to the cost of the incentive. What value will participants place on the incentive? Will the perceived value be a sufficiently high motivator?

When money is used as an incentive for participating in multiple interviews, escalating the amount for each successive interview or giving a bonus for completing all interviews may be more effective than a flat rate. For some, nonmonetary incentives, either as an alternative or an addition to money, may be more effective in encouraging participation. This is especially important when the purpose of the program is to pilot education programs in other communities where monetary incentives may not be available. Once having taken part in the intervention, the participant should be motivated enough to attend the group or talk with the health care provider or drug counselor without an incentive.

Ideally, incentives should not only be meaningful to the target population, but should have a potentially reinforcing effect on the target behavior and should be relevant to the intervention content. For example, distributing keychains that hold condoms can serve as a potent reminder to use condoms for every sexual act. Table 9.1 illustrates how some prevention programs tailored incentives to different populations.

Table 9.1. Incentives by Targeted Population

Population	Incentives used	Source
Gay men	Rugby shirts with study logo	GMHC (Mantell *et al.*, 1989a)
	Safer sex kits	GMHC (Mantell *et al.*, 1989a)
	Bandanas with safer sex messages written on them	Ohio State Department of Health (B. Harris, personal communication, 1988)
Sex workers	Self-defense training; make-up lessons; storefront to "hang out in," shower and refreshments	ADAPT (Y. Serrano, personal communication, 1988)
	Medical evaluations in hotel rooms in San Francisco	AWARE (Cohen, Alexander, & Wofsy, 1988)
	Prizes to high scorers on AIDS knowledge tests	CAL-PEP
Inner-city women	Child care services	New York Department of Health
	Transportation	(Mantell *et al.*, 1995b)
	Stipend	
Injection drug users	Coupons to expedite admission to drug treatment	New Jersey Department of Health (Jackson & Rotkiewicz, 1987)
	Graduation ceremonies and certificates of completion	GMHC, Project HEART (Mantell *et al.*, 1989b)
	Case management services to bridge drug and medical treatment	Needle Exchange Programs (C. Eaton, personal communication, 1989; Shulman, Mantell, Eaton, & Sorrell, 1990)

Disadvantages

The use of incentives can have some methodological effects. First, they introduce a source of bias in that people who participate in programs that distribute incentives may differ from those willing to participate in a study without an extrinsic reward. For example, participants may be more knowledgeable or sensitized to the issue of HIV/AIDS. Second, incentives may create among participants a feeling of having to repay the interviewer or researcher with the "correct" or socially desirable answer or behavior. Third, among some closed communities (e.g., clients of methadone maintenance treatment programs), groups of "professional intervention participants" may be created. This group, in effect, "sells" their participation to the highest bidder, further restricting the generalizability of results.

The effects of different monetary incentives on retaining participants in an intervention can be tested with a randomized design. For example, participants could be randomly allocated to one of four conditions: (1) a flat payment, (2) escalating payments, (3) a flat payment with a large bonus for the last assessment, and (4) no payment. Differences in group follow-up rates would be monitored.

INDIVIDUAL- VERSUS COMMUNITY-LEVEL INTERVENTION

Since the beginning of the HIV epidemic, individual-level change directed to individuals and small groups has been the major thrust of interventions to reduce high-risk sexual and drug-related behaviors. The relative dearth of community-level evaluation to determine overall behavioral change (Kelly, 1994) is not surprising since community-level intervention development in AIDS is still in a relatively embryonic stage. Calls for large-scale mobilization initiatives on the order of the "War against Drugs," which involve the dedication of huge public health disease intervention technology resource transfer, to combat the spread of HIV have been put forth (Kelly *et al.*, 1993; Cohen, 1993). These strategies in themselves, however, will probably do little to control HIV. Rather, a communitarian approach, which seeks to empower and mobilize communities to undertake community-centered HIV health promotion initiatives (Isbell, 1993), may be more appropriate.

Only over the past 8 years has there been a thrust toward community-level population-based prevention in AIDS, for example, the CDC's five-city AIDS Community Demonstration and Women and AIDS Demonstration Projects (O'Reilly & Higgins, 1991) and NIDA's Community Demonstration Projects targeted to injection drug users (IDUs) and female sex partners of IDUs (McCoy & Inciardi, 1993). Its precedence has been established in public health programs for cardiovascular risk reduction and smoking cessation (Maccoby, Farquhar, Wood, & Alexander, 1977; McAlister, Puska, Salomen, & Koskela, 1982; Farquhar & Maccoby, 1984; COMMIT Research Group, 1995a,b). These interventions encompass more than information transmission, e.g., media campaigns to increase community awareness of HIV vaccines or zidovudine for pregnant women. They can play a pivotal role in HIV prevention by promoting norms for the social acceptability of condom use, motivating the use of bleach to clean injection equipment, facilitating access to early treatment, and encouraging compliance with therapy.

While the designs of an individual- and community-level intervention may be similar, their application is different. Kelly and colleagues (Kelly *et al.*, 1993; Kelly, 1994) classified extant HIV behavioral intervention research into three categories. We collapsed this typology into two major classifications: (1) face-to-face contact with individuals or groups; and (2) focus on community-wide change. At the individual level, interventions targeted to groups differ from those directed to the individual in that group dynamics, role modeling, and pressure to conform to peer norms can be used to influence individuals' initiation and maintenance of risk-reduction behavior.

Table 9.2 characterizes the constellation of cardinal features of individual- and community-level interventions. Interventions targeted to the individual or small groups are at the individual level, usually with an individual-level analysis. In a community-level intervention, a community or population is targeted, and the community is the unit of analysis. With individual-level interventions, a relatively small group of individuals are reached, and behavioral change is expected to materialize in a short period of time.

Table 9.2. Hallmarks of Individual- and Community-Level Interventions

Dimension	Individual level	Community level
Target population	Small audience	Large audience
Unit of analysis	Individuals and small single- or multiple-session groups	Populations and communities
Timeframe	Short-term (impact)	Long-term (outcome)
Outcome indicators	Single or multiple indicators: Increased condom use Increased use of sterile drug paraphernalia Reduced use of injection drugs Reduced episodes of STDs (e.g., gonorrhea and syphilis)	Single or multiple indicators: Trends in condom sales Increased number of drug treatment slots Increased condom use during vaginal, anal, and oral sex Social norms promoting condom use Increased access to condoms (e.g., vending machines, schools) Reduced incidence and prevalence of HIV infection and other STDs over time Increased use of syringe exchange program Increased use of AIDS hotlines
Intent of intervention	Individual change Knowledge, attitudes, and behavior (e.g., compliance with STD treatment)	Community-wide change in knowledge, attitudes, and behavior Influence social norms (e.g., promoting condom use in brothels) Community empowerment
Setting	Single or multiple venues Clinic, drug treatment center, family planning center, community-based organization, churches	Multiple venues Housing project, neighborhood, schools, public transportation stations

(continued)

Table 9.2. (*Continued*)

Dimension	Individual level	Community level
Components of intervention	Single approach is typical, but multiple approaches may be employed	Multiple approaches
Intervention modalities	One-on-one Single event intervention Workshops	Outreach Small media Mass media
Intervention content (how the content of the intervention is implemented will determine if it is individual level and/or community level)	Counseling/contact notification assistance Problem-solving skills AIDS hotlines Peer support HIV counseling and testing Counselor/peer training Theatre Community forums/town meetings Health fairs Videos Peer outreach Information dissemination through radio and TV PSA campaigns, billboards, and posters Syringe exchange	
Community involvement	Not required, although community members and peer opinion leaders may be solicited	Comprehensive strategy with involvement of multiple community sectors and organizations (e.g., providers, worksite) Mobilization of communities to take on AIDS prevention as a mission and spearhead prevention activities Community-wide intervention blitz Use of formal or informal role models to model specific behaviors Involvement in high-profile community groups, key informants, and gatekeepers
Date collection strategies	Single or multiple	Usually multiple
Cost	Ranges from relatively inexpensive to expensive	Labor-intensive Always expensive
Evaluation strategy	Impact evaluation	Outcome evaluation

Community-wide interventions aim for long-term changes in social norms and behaviors and are targeted to large groups—populations or communities. Often, changes in community members' behavior can be more easily measured in small geographically contained cities with a relatively stable population insulated from more metropolitan areas (Kelly, 1994). A longitudinal cohort approach in which both intervention and comparison communities are followed over time is usually employed. There is also a reliance on natural channels within the indigenous community to provide information and skills (Hays & Peterson, 1994). A social diffusion model (Rogers, 1983), described in

Chapter 8, has been the dominant model for using social networks and social modeling techniques to promote adoption of behavioral change.

Community-level intervention often entails multiple channels and ways to reach the target population. The venue for delivering an AIDS community prevention program may be within an identifiable location such as a church or school. However, more transient, changing communities, where people come together for some reason, e.g., radio listeners, transportation carriers, and the undomiciled, are also potential venues for directing community intervention. These venues are particularly fitting for delivering messages to a built-in audience who would not necessarily seek information about HIV risk reduction.

There are several limitations to community-level intervention. They are expensive and require time before effects can be seen. Multiple strategies and sources of data collection are central to a community-level HIV preventive intervention (McAlister *et al.*, 1982). Validity is of concern, since secular trends, shifting social norms, and other extraneous factors may confound intervention outcomes (Rothenberg, 1993). However, with a randomized community trial that uses matched pairs of intervention and control communities, these threats can be reduced (as discussed in Chapter 5).

COMMUNITY-LEVEL INTERVENTION VERSUS COMMUNITY-LEVEL EVALUATION

A distinction between community-level preventive intervention and community-level evaluation must be made. An intervention can be community-wide, but evaluation still may be at the individual level only, community level only, or both. Impact evaluation is directed toward individual-level interventions. In contrast, outcome evaluation is directed toward community-level interventions. Community-level evaluation of normative change should be carefully planned and measured rather than evaluation of an incidental outcome or a series of unrelated interventions.

For example, if eight AIDS organizations planned, implemented, and evaluated eight independent park outreach programs, intervention and evaluation are not at the community-level. On the other hand, implementation and evaluation of a *Love in the Time of AIDS* campaign (W. Badillo, 1994, personal communication), featuring coordinated park outreaches conducted by a consortium of eight organizations, is at the community-level. In the first case, the cumulative effects of eight concurrent but independent outreach efforts would be assessed, while in the second case the coordinated effort of a single, multilevel intervention (a case of the whole being greater than the sum of its parts) would be assessed. Hence, it is important to keep in mind that community-level intervention is not simply the individual intervention repeated many times in a community. Rather, it is a comprehensive, population-based planned and targeted strategy for community change.

INTERVENTION MODALITIES

As noted in Table 9.2, the content or method of the intervention is neither intrinsically individual nor community level. It is how the method is incorporated in the study design and how the intervention as a whole is evaluated that determine whether the unit of analysis is the individual or the community. For example, if an AIDS hotline is established to increase awareness about HIV/AIDS and decrease high-risk behaviors among the callers, then this would be an individual-level intervention, with evaluation at that level. Evaluation techniques include postcall interviews with the callers or questionnaires mailed to the callers following the intervention. However, if the AIDS hotline was part of a community-wide campaign to increase AIDS awareness and foster norms of safer sex, then the intervention would be community level and evaluated as such.

In this section, we review some popularly used intervention modalities and provide illustrations of them. It must be kept in mind that the content of the interventions is not limited to the individual- or community-level modality; given a different study design, they would be interchangeable. It is only for the purpose of discussion that the intervention content is listed under individual- or community-level modality.

Individual-Level Interventions

The individual-level intervention, especially one-on-one, single-event, and workshop modalities, has been the most popular among AIDS health educators.

One-on-One Interventions

One-on-one interventions are those in which the individual is exposed to HIV-related education by the health educator in a dyadic relationship. Examples of these types of interventions include HIV counseling and testing, notification assistance, peer intervention, tabling (the setting up of tables with information about HIV prevention and care in a community), AIDS hotlines, and HIV prevention technology.

Counseling and Testing Activities. HIV risk-reduction counseling and testing at anonymous sites, hospitals, and doctors' offices, family planning clinics, TB clinics, drug treatment facilities, STD clinics, colleges, and prisons is an important area requiring program evaluation. As an intervention strategy, HIV counseling and testing has focused on both behavioral change and early detection of HIV infection. There have been relatively few attempts to evaluate these programs. Surveys of men and women receiving these services can provide important baseline data on sociodemographics, HIV-related knowledge, and the prevalence of high-risk sexual and drug injection behaviors. This information in turn can be used to target both the type and level of prevention education as well as those health and social services needed by the population. A sample form for recording information from people seeking HIV counseling and testing at various sites is shown in Fig. 9.1.

Evaluation of HIV counseling and testing programs can also provide information about trends in testing practices, motivations for being tested (and retested), why people return for notification of serostatus, whether knowledge of serostatus promotes behavioral change, and personal and situational characteristics of tested individuals. Research questions may include the following: Since therapeutic benefits of getting tested have been stressed, has there been an increase in the number of people seeking HIV testing? What proportion of people have been tested previously? Why are people seeking repeat

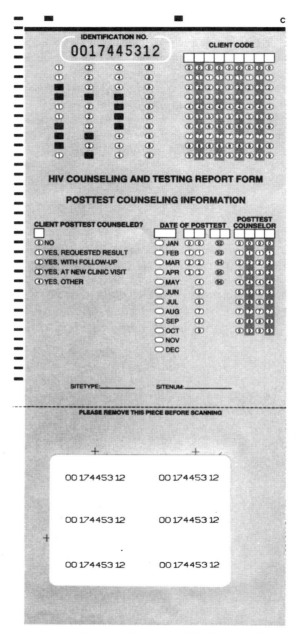

Figure 9.1. HIV counseling and testing report form. (From U.S. Centers for Disease Control and Prevention.)

Figure 9.1. (*Continued*)

testing? Has Magic Johnson's public disclosure of being HIV-infected led to people reducing their high-risk sexual behaviors?

Health educators and clinicians should also be clear about what information cannot be provided by evaluation of an HIV counseling and testing program. HIV seroprevalence rates especially those reported from anonymous counseling and testing (ACT) sites, do not provide an accurate assessment of the true rate of new infections in a community, since the tested individuals may not come from the ACT site community. HIV counseling sessions are difficult to evaluate because of the brevity of the intervention. What outcomes should be expected from these limited counseling interventions? For example, is it realistic to expect that pregnant women who learn during a brief counseling session that they are infected will terminate their pregnancy? Should counseling of infected women influence their decisions about future pregnancies? Client anonymity also constrains an evaluator's ability to contact clients for follow-up assessments.

Intervention/control group designs in which counseling is withheld generally are not used in the evaluation of HIV counseling and testing programs because it would be unethical to do so. Evaluation strategies have consisted of process measures, qualitative data, pretest–posttest designs with one follow-up assessment, longitudinal pretest–posttest designs with multiple follow-up assessments, and experimental–comparison group designs in which the counseling method or intensity or level of group counseling are varied.

The National Research Council Panel on the Evaluation of AIDS Interventions (Coyle e *al.*, 1991) recommends that data be collected from multiple sources, including administrators and staff from testing sites, clients, groups that engage in high-risk behavior, and independent observers, to evaluate five dimensions of service delivery:

- Adequacy of the counseling and testing protocol (e.g., confidentiality, waiting time for test results, security of linkage between counseling and testing, disclosure of test results, and, among the HIV-infected, partner notification).
- Adequacy of the counseling provided (support, risk assessment, and provision of accurate information about HIV transmission and risk-reduction techniques).
- Proportion of clients that complete the full protocol.
- Accessibility to services.
- Types of barriers to accessing services and completing counseling and testing activities.

They also point to the importance of considering the setting in which services are delivered, since individuals who are counseled and tested in family planning, drug treatment, or STD clinics may be less motivated to return for posttest counseling and test results because they attended the clinics for non-HIV-related reasons.

The impact of counseling intensity on behavior change could be assessed by randomly assigning half of the subjects to a five-session counseling intervention and the other half to the standard counseling intervention (which typically consists of one session). With captive or closed populations such as methadone or drug-free treatment cohorts, different approaches to HIV counseling and testing can be assessed. One approach would be to assess the effects of two types of subject motivation on behavioral and psychological outcomes by comparing a client group enrolled in a counseling and testing study (program-motivated) with a group that seeks counseling and testing on its own (client-motivated); alternatively, the effects of offering counseling and testing as part of an agency's routine intake process versus client-initiated counseling and testing can be compared (Rugg, MacGowan, Stark, & Swanson, 1991).

The impact of a single-session, postpartum HIV counseling session for HIV-infected women in Nairobi, Kenya, was evaluated by a pretest–posttest design, with comparison group as part of a study of the relationship between maternal HIV infection and pregnancy outcomes, as described in Example 9.2. Global indicators, such as

---

Example 9.2. Counseling HIV-Infected Women in Nairobi, Kenya

Intervention Description

Women with an adverse pregnancy outcome (low birth weight or stillbirth) and a control group of women who delivered normal birth weight infants were recruited from a hospital-based postpartum clinic. Physical and gynecological exams and one counseling session 7 to 10 days postpartum were offered. At the counseling session, women were informed of their HIV status and counseled about risk-reduction measures. HIV-positive women were counseled about the need to inform their spouses of their diagnosis and to return to the clinic in 2 weeks for additional counseling. Condoms were distributed and other methods of family planning were encouraged.

Evaluation Strategy

A pretest–posttest design with comparison group was used. Impact evaluation of the counseling session consisted of matching by pregnancy outcome, 94 asymptomatic HIV-positive women with 94 of their noninfected counterparts 1 year postpartum. Among the HIV-positive women with a known address, only 51 could be contacted and 24 returned for the 1-year follow-up visit. Among the seronegative women, 56 could be contacted and 33 returned for the 1-year follow-up. Social, medical, and obstetrical events and contraceptive practices over the 1 year were documented.

The "success" of the counseling session was assessed by:

- Whether seropositive women had informed their partner of their serostatus.
- Whether knowledge of a positive serostatus had influenced reproductive behaviors (e.g., limited family size as reflected by the pregnancy rate).
- Increased condom use and other methods of contraception (e.g., pill).

Results

Only 37% of the HIV-positive women notified their partner of their serostatus. There were no statistically significant differences between the HIV-positive and HIV-negative women with respect to pregnancy rates.

(SOURCE: Temmerman et al., 1990.)

reduction in unprotected anal and vaginal intercourse and reduction in new HIV infection rates, can also be used to assess behavioral change.

Many ACT sites offer an intense one-on-one education intervention as well as testing services. For example, the pretest counseling program at the New York City Department of Health's ACT sites provides extensive education in risk reduction, transmission modes, general AIDS information, and understanding the HIV test. In addition, risk assessment, via review of drug and sex history, is performed as well as general health planning and resource referral/utilization. Similar information is reinforced during posttest counseling.

Process evaluation can provide information about the effectiveness and consistency of service delivery. Examples of process indicators are:

- The number of clients receiving counseling.
- The number of counseled clients who were tested.
- Number of counseling sessions held and length of each session.
- Whether counseling and testing session is the first session or a repeat one.
- Sociodemographic characteristics of clients.
- Counselor characteristics.
- Client satisfaction with the program.
- Staff satisfaction with the program.

Qualitative methods include focus groups, personal interviews with clients and staff, observation of clients in the waiting room, and observation of the counseling intervention.

By collecting an extensive database, program planners will be better able to chart the epidemic and target audiences for community-based education. Outcome evaluation of the counseling and testing intervention can serve to strengthen and test the efficacy of the educational model.

In addition to raising ethical issues, the use of control groups in the evaluation of HIV counseling and testing programs may make the evaluation of these programs a challenge. First, it is difficult to disentangle the effects of the counseling process from knowledge of test results and the notification process and, likewise, increased awareness of AIDS as a result of being tested from disclosure of HIV status. Second, variations in HIV counseling and testing interventions by site can make comparative analysis of findings difficult. Third, as with any quasi-experimental intervention, the sample size must be large enough to provide adequate power to detect statistically significant differences between experimental and comparison groups. Selection bias may also operate in that subjects who enroll in counseling and testing studies may be more predisposed to changing high-risk behaviors than those who do not enroll or who are counseled and tested as part of an agency's routine intake assessment. This source of confounding can be adjusted for by controlling for HIV serostatus and adding several comparison groups—"never-tested," refusers, those who accept the offer but do not actively seek counseling and testing—and comparing their HIV risk behaviors (Rugg *et al.*, 1991). Finally, evaluations conducted with samples of low-risk participants may underestimate the true effects of counseling and testing on changing risk behavior.

Certain subsets of clients may be reluctant to seek HIV counseling and testing services provided through traditional means. Mobile vans set up as miniclinics to provide counseling and testing services may be an effective way to reach those people who will not otherwise come to alternate or confidential counseling and testing sites. A roving clinic concept entails taking programs to communities on their own terms. Such outreach efforts have already been put into practice for IDUs who are not otherwise in treatment (S. Tross, personal communication) and for patrons of gay bars (Miller, 1989). Similar mobile counseling and testing outreach at roadside rest stops, where men frequently have sex with men, has been funded in New Jersey. Evaluation of these nontraditional programs can determine the degree to which outreach efforts at these sites are effective in reaching the population, changing high-risk sexual behaviors, and maintaining behavioral change.

Finally, population-based surveys of the general population in specific neighborhoods that include nonusers of the service can provide important information about potential barriers to accessing services (Coyle *et al.*, 1991). In this case, assessment is at the community level.

Voluntary HIV Contact Notification Assistance Programs.   Specific quantitative and qualitative measures can be used to gauge the success of partner referral or notification programs, as shown in Table 9.3.

Peer Educator Programs.   Peer educator programs have become increasingly popular as an HIV prevention strategy. Educators are recruited from the ranks of the target population to teach their cohorts how to think about their sexual and drug use practices and reduce their risks for HIV infection. The intent is for these community opinion leaders to change normative beliefs and behaviors through peer influence

Table 9.3.   Criteria for Evaluating Partner Notification Programs[a]

Quantitative measures
   Number of index persons enrolled in the program
   Numbers of partners identified
   Sociodemographic characteristics of the participants
   Number of partners notified and counseled
   HIV seroprevalence of partners
   Number of partners who agree to be tested
   Number of partners who enroll in community prevention programs
   Program costs
Qualitative measures
   Participants' satisfaction with the program
   Participants' compliance with safer sex guidelines
   Program acceptability
   Adequacy and intensity of staff training
   Adequacy of participant follow-up

[a]Adapted from the World Health Organization (1989).

Table 9.4.   Selected Criteria for Evaluating
the Impact of a Peer Educator Program

- Changes in clients' HIV-related knowledge, attitudes, and behaviors over time
- Client satisfaction with the one-to-one or group educational session
- Peer educator satisfaction with the intervention
- Number of initial and repeated sessions with clients
- Number of client referrals to health and social service agencies
- Number of individual sessions and groups held
- Number and types of literature distributed

motivation and social feedback. Criteria by which to gauge the effectiveness of a peer educator program are noted in Table 9.4.

Closed communities, such as homeless shelters, schools, and drug treatment centers, are ideal sites to implement a peer education program. In these instances, leaders are readily identifiable and are role models in the health education of their cohorts. One such program was instituted in three homeless shelters in Brooklyn, New York. The program, Project REACH stands for Residents Educating About Community Health. Its general philosophy is that training residents in the shelters to provide public health information (e.g., HIV/AIDS education, tuberculosis) tailored to the needs of the homeless would be the most effective means of decreasing the incidence of HIV transmission and increasing general health awareness and practices (e.g., increased use of condoms, increased HIV testing).

The program has been in effect for 4 years and the peer educators make over 13,000 contacts per year. These contacts are made through the provision of group educational programs, tabling events, outreach in the community, "in-reach" in the shelters, one-on-one educational sessions, and other educationally based interventions. Systematic evaluation of the impact this program has had on the shelter communities served has not yet been performed (DiVittis & Badillo, 1995).

AIDS Education Tabling Events.   These events entail the distribution of HIV-related information from tables in public places (e.g., street corners, at health fairs, airports, train stations, in schools, community centers, post offices, bars, and gay bathhouses). Information is given in a brief interaction between the health educator staffing the table and the consumer who either takes information in the form of brochures, or condoms, or gets his or her information from the health educator in a brief interaction. This type of intervention warrants evaluation. A sample assessment form used by New York City's GMHC is shown in Table 9.5.

With a data base form, potentially vital information—audience characteristics (ethnicity, gender, and age), number of volunteers and volunteer hours, number and kinds of educational brochures distributed, content of audience questions, audience level of knowledge, and structural factors (location of tabling event, weather), to name a few—can be monitored and evaluated. The value of this type of process evaluation is that it provides program planners with an assessment of the informational needs of the constituents of various communities.

Table 9.5. Assessment Form for AIDS Prevention Tabling Events[a]

Date: _____   Location: _____
Indoor: _____   Outdoor: _____   Weather: _____
Volunteers: _____   Hours worked: _____   Total: _____

_____   _____   _____

_____   _____   _____

_____   _____   _____

_____   _____   _____

No. of hours at table site: _____   From: _____   To: _____   Total: _____
Audience reached:
1. Ethnic content: White: _____   Black: _____   Hispanic: _____   Asian: _____   Other: _____
2. Sex: Male: _____   Female: _____
3. Age range: 1–10: _____   10–18: _____   19–25: _____   25–35: _____
            35–50: _____   50+: _____
Content of question and conversation:
1. HIV testing information   _____   Support/reassurance   _____
2. Symptoms   _____   Non-AIDS related   _____
3. Transmission   _____   Other   _____
4. Safer sex   _____
5. Treatment/new drugs   _____
6. General AIDS information _____
Comments:

Basic knowledge about AIDS of the population at the table site:
Very informed _____   Somewhat informed _____
Not very informed _____   Not at all informed _____
Misinformed _____
General response to this GMHC AIDS-information table:
Great _____   Good _____   Fair _____   Poor _____   Hostile/aggressive _____
Number of respondents:

[a]From Gay Men's Health Crisis (1989), with permission.

In addition to the process evaluation of tabling events, impact evaluation is also needed. An impact evaluation would assess the degree to which the information distributed has effected behavior change. Further, with ethnographic methods, the impact of health information disseminated through literature distribution on the norms of the communities in question can be ascertained.

AIDS Hotlines. These provide means of dispersing information about HIV/AIDS in brief, usually anonymous, interactions between the operator (e.g., health/peer educator) and the caller. Information can include direct public health information regarding transmission/prevention and referrals to HIV counseling and testing sites. Hotlines are often difficult to evaluate given the brief and anonymous nature of the interaction.

A survey that gauges callers' perceptions of their satisfaction with the hotline (in terms of making appropriate referrals and providing emotional reassurance and information) is one means of determining both quality and effectiveness. Measurement is confined, however, to the time immediately following a given call. To maintain anonymity, the counseling or referral portion of the call could be handled by one hotline worker and the consequent evaluation by another staff member or volunteer. This strategy is limited. Outcome measures, such as the hotline's effect on the caller's attitudes or behaviors, cannot be assessed. The script and questionnaire used by GMHC to evaluate their AIDS hotline are shown in Table 9.6.

Hotlines can also be evaluated in terms of the number and length of calls, reasons for calling, and, if possible, sociodemographics of the caller. Data bases are necessary to document this information. The GMHC Hotline maintained a descriptive, anonymous survey of calls, by shift, by volunteer to help monitor trends in service utilization. A tally that included general headings such as gender, sexual behavior (e.g., gay, heterosexual, etc.), type of call (local, long distance, TDD), population (e.g., people with AIDS, IDU, etc.), content (e.g., testing, transmission prevention), and referral/action taken and duration of call in minutes was taken for each call received. Given that calls were anonymous, descriptive information about the caller was not always available (Dozier, 1989).

Another method of evaluating an AIDS education and counseling hotline is to use a simulation procedure (Kosecoff & Fink, 1976). This technique entails writing scripts of scenarios that reflect the needs of typical hotline callers. The "confederates" going to make the simulated calls must be trained to deliver the script and complete an evaluation form. The evaluation form can be used to code hotline volunteers' responses by what is essential, acceptable, and unacceptable information as well as the caller's perceptions of the empathy and clarity of the volunteer's response. An example of a simulated call in which the caller wants information is provided in Example 9.3.

HIV Prevention Technology.   With the ever-changing technology in HIV/AIDS prevention, intervention and evaluation strategies become intertwined to arrive at the most effective means of meeting the needs of communities for these prevention products. One such recent example is the creation of the vaginal pouch, or "female condom." Given the newness of this technology, special care is needed in the marketing, training, and presentation of this new barrier method option for women. Mantell, Karim, and Scheepers (1996) developed a multiphase intervention using tenets from the diffusion of innovation model (Rogers, 1983) and social learning theory (Bandura, 1977a) as the theoretical underpinning. A "train the trainers" approach was used to train South African health care providers in how to introduce female barriers methods into public health clinics and to counsel women about a range of alternatives to the male condom and to increase negotiation skills.

The first phase of the intervention consisted of training the health care providers. Efficacy of training was determined using a pretest–posttest study design, targeting changes in trainees' knowledge and attitudes.

Phase two included process and impact evaluation methods. Implementation evaluation focusing on the replicability of training and the intervention model in various sites will be conducted. Some key indicators include degree to which health care providers felt the training prepared them for the clinic implementation phase, average number of clients per week counseled about the methods, number of female and male condoms distributed to both new and continuing clients, and providers' and clients' satisfaction

Table 9.6. Evaluation Tool for Assessment of GMHC's AIDS Hotline

Script for hotline counselor who transfers calls to the volunteer who will do the survey.

Once you have fully responded to the caller's request, say the following, or paraphrase in your own words:
"I hope we have been able to help you. There are some people who are going through the same changes as you. In order to better serve them, we are trying to improve the hotline. Could you answer a few questions? It would require only a minute or two of your time."

If the caller says *Yes*:
"I am going to turn you over to our interviewer." (Give the phone to the interviewer.)

If the caller says *No*:
"Thank you for your call. Please use our number in the future."

Script for hotline counselor who interviews the caller:
"Thank you for agreeing to answer our survey. I am going to ask you seven questions. Please answer on a scale of 1 to 5 with 1 being *not at all* and 5 being *totally*. [Adminster the survey. Remember to indicate the date, sex of caller, and type of peer counseling (reinforcement support = S; education = E; referral = R) for each call.] "Thank you for your time. Please use our number in the future."

Date: _____ Sex of caller: _____ Type of peer counseling provided: _____

Instructions to interviewer: For each of the following questions, please ask the caller to rate his/her response according to the rating scale, and circle the number for each response.

1. Did you get what you needed from the counselor?

1	2	3	4	5
not at all	a little	halfway	mostly	totally

2. Did the counselor spend enough time with you?

1	2	3	4	5
not at all	a little	halfway	mostly	totally

3. Do you plan to follow through with the counselor's suggestions?

1	2	3	4	5
not at all	a little	halfway	mostly	totally

4. Were you comfortable with the attitude of the counselor?

1	2	3	4	5
not at all	a little	halfway	mostly	totally

5. Were your expectations of talking on the hotline fulfilled?

1	2	3	4	5
not at all	a little	halfway	mostly	totally

6. Do you feel better after having spoken with the counselor?

1	2	3	4	5
not at all	a little	halfway	mostly	totally

7. Do you have any additional comments?

_____

_____

*a*From Dozier (1989), with permission.

Example 9.3. Simulated AIDS Hotline Call

Background

 The caller is a 23-year-old Latino man who has AIDS as a result of long-standing injection of drugs and sharing needles. He has a 21-year-old wife who also has AIDS and two young children, aged 1 and 3. The youngest child was born infected with HIV. The manager of the caller's apartment building has told the caller he and his family can no longer live in the building.

Script

 My doctor told me I had AIDS. It's been 1 year now. My wife and youngest daughter are in the hospital now. My wife has been sick for months. The doctors just told me that my wife and baby have the virus. When my neighbors found out about my situation, they told the owner of my apartment building. The owner, he told me that I had to get out, that he was afraid I would give the virus to others in the building. I don't know what to do. Can you help me?

---

with training and educational materials. Key benchmarks for impact evaluation include acceptance of methods by clients and their sexual partners, clients' ability to use the female condom correctly, increase in the proportion of new clients using the female condom over time, and increase in the proportion of women maintaining use of the female condom.

 Phase three of the intervention will be to implement a "train the trainers" approach among female and male community leaders. Six-month assessments are planned, focusing on the effectiveness of the intervention using benchmarks such as consistency of condom use, acceptance of the methods, and self-efficacy in sexual decision-making skills. The impact evaluation will assess the success of the application of the diffusion of innovation model. Women entering the clinic will be asked where they learned of the services offered, thus mapping the informal referral process.

Single-Event Interventions

 The single-event intervention is a group-oriented presentation that occurs one time only. Examples of these types of interventions include theater/drama, video presentations, and home risk-reduction parties.

 Theater/Drama. This is a popular and innovative forum for AIDS education, similar to psychodrama, that draws on role-playing techniques to impart HIV prevention messages. The audience actively participates in the educational process. As a medium, theater appeals to a broad and versatile audience of different ages and educational levels and can be effective in reaching people who might not attend HIV prevention programs through traditional means. While some theater companies employ professional actors, others train and employ people from the local community.

A series of skits or role plays that depict a problem or issue, such as negotiation around condom use, alternatives to sexual intercourse, and deciding whether to undergo HIV testing, are enacted. In some theater interventions, conflict dilemmas are improvised and the audience participates. The action of the play is stopped at the point of crisis. Members of the audience are invited to come on the stage to act out the scene in a different manner. The professional actors then respond to the way in which the amateur actor plays the situation. The play is stopped again and another member of the audience is invited to play the skit. After several iterations, audience discussion follows. Since there is more than one way to resolve a dilemma, the various problem-solving strategies derived by audience members provide an effective peer means for teaching people new options.

For example, Teen Teatro, in which teens have been trained as community peer AIDS educators, used the medium of a play to increase awareness of HIV transmission and promote risk reduction among Latino youth in Los Angeles County. Following the 20- to 30-minute play, the teen actors/educators conducted a 20- to 30-minute rap session with the audience.

Several strategies were used to evaluate this theater project. First, the script for the play was submitted to a community review process and field tested with community leaders and community-based organizations (CBOs). An evaluation form, which focused on the messages in the script, its methods, and effectiveness and those in the follow-up discussion, was distributed at the end of the audience discussion. This process evaluation resulted in useful information about how to reach the target audience, the appropriateness of specific words, and the use of slang, which topics to emphasize, and the ideal length of the play. The field test evaluation form used during the community review process is shown in Table 9.7.

Second, once the review process was completed, evaluation of the theater/discussion intervention consisted of process and outcome measures, as shown in Table 9.8. Impact evaluation of another theater intervention to reduce adolescents' risk of AIDS and other STDs and prevent pregnancy is described in Example 9.4.

As with the Teen Teatro intervention discussed earlier, changes in behavior cannot be assessed with this type of intervention. Subjects' anonymous completion of the questionnaires would make it difficult to track them several months after the performance to ascertain the correspondence between reported intentions and behaviors.

Other researchers have taken advantage of "natural" theatrical events and evaluated audience reactions to plays about AIDS. In a university community, two performances of William Hoffman's play, *As Is*, about a gay man with AIDS, were evaluated with a preperformance–postperformance design (Probart, 1989). With the postperformance evaluation conducted immediately after the performance, impact assessment was limited to changes in AIDS-related knowledge and beliefs. Because of the difficulty of conducting personal interviews before or after the performance, self-administered questionnaires were used and distributed in booklet form. After the audience was seated,

Table 9.7. East Los Angeles Rape Hotline Inc.
Teen Teatro AIDS Prevention Project (Teen TAPP)[a]

Field Test Evaluation Form

Name: _____

Agency affiliation: _____

1. Do you feel the teatro presentation (play and narration) addressed the following topics? Why or why not?
   HIV transmission: _____
   AIDS prevention: _____
   Correction of myths: _____

2. Do you think the following aspects are appropriate for delivery to a Latino youth audience?
   Linguistic relevance: _____
   Cultural relevance: _____
   Literacy level (age appropriateness): _____
   Length of presentation: _____

3. Do you feel that the presentation effectively communicates to a teen audience member the *urgency* of making AIDS risk-reduction behavioral changes? Why or why not?

4. How well did the actors encourage participation from the audience?
   _____

5. What did you like most about the presentation?
   _____

6. What did you like least about the presentation?
   _____

7. Additional comments
   _____

8. We have tentatively scheduled the Teen TAPP community preview for a later date in _____. In order that we can assure that a broad cross-section of agencies dealing with Latino youth are present, please list below 5–7 agencies, contact persons, and phone numbers that we may add to our invitation mailing list.
   _____

[a]From US Conference of Mayors (1989), with permission.

Table 9.8. Process and Outcome Evaluation Measures
for Teen Teatro AIDS Education Program[a]

Process measures
    Number of performances scheduled
    Number of people attending performances
    Number of organizations asking for a second performance
    Number of actors/peer educators trained
    Number of staff review sessions held
    Number of advisory committee meetings held
Outcome measures
    Pretest–posttest measures of knowledge and attitudes about HIV transmission and prevention methods
    Number of phone calls to the Spanish language AIDS hotline associated with the performance
    Staff review of the "rap" sessions that followed performance, especially the types of questions asked that
        should have been covered in the performance.

[a]From US Conference of Mayors (1989), with permission.

Example 9.4. New Image Teen Theater Intervention, New York

Evaluation Design

Pretest–posttest design focused on impact evaluation. Outcomes of interest were: (1) willingness to and comfort in communicating with adults and other teens about sex; (2) intentions to use birth control; (3) intentions to protect themselves from STDs by using condoms; (4) intentions to delay sexual intercourse; (5) sexual knowledge; and (6) positive and negative affect felt during the performance (on the posttest only). Questionnaires were distributed as the teens entered the auditorium at schools and churches. The pretests were collected prior to the start of the performance and the posttests were completed and collected immediately after the performance. Following completion of the posttest, a discussion was held. Participation was anonymous.

Sample

One hundred forty-three male and female adolescents aged 13–17 years of diverse ethnic backgrounds.

Results

Evaluation showed that, following the theater performance, the teens reported greater willingness to discuss sexual issues, increased intention to use birth control, and greater sexual knowledge; mean differences in pre- and posttest scores were modest, however. There were no statistically significant differences in comfort level in talking about sex, intention to protect themselves from STDs, and intention to delay sexual intercourse. The replication of these findings across seven diverse audiences enhances their generalizability to other groups of youth.

(SOURCE: Hillman, Hovell, Williams, Hofstetter, & Burdyshaw, 1991.)

---

the director of the production asked them to complete the first part of the booklet before the play began and the second part afterward. A container was provided for audience members to deposit their questionnaires as they left the theater.

Results of the evaluation indicated a slight, but statistically significant, decrease in knowledge scores at posttest (from 17.5 to 16.6). This was probably attributed to the high knowledge scores at pretest (ceiling effect). Also, fear generated by the drama may have accounted for the minimal change. Changes in AIDS-related beliefs, measured by tolerance of persons with HIV infection, were not statistically significant. With this type of evaluation, assessment of behavioral change is not possible.

Another innovative medium related to live performance theater is the use of puppetry for HIV prevention education. Puppetry appeals to a diverse adult, adolescent, and child audience, can deliver prevention messages in a nonthreatening manner, and easily can be understood by people with little formal education. "Puppets against AIDS" was used to educate a variety of South African cultural groups (Skinner, Metcalf, Seager, de Swardt, & Laubscher, 1991). Evaluation of the puppet show consisted of two phases: (1) a content analysis of a video recording of the puppet show conducted by a five-person multidisciplinary group according to a priori criteria; and (2) an impact evaluation with a pretest–posttest design. Impact evaluation aimed to:

- Assess the impact of the show on audience knowledge of HIV infection/AIDS and intentions regarding short-term risk-reduction behaviors.
- Determine whether the educational messages were understood by the audience.
- Assess the cultural sensitivity of the content of the puppet show.

A convenience sample of 208 people participated in both the pre- and posttest interview and another 96 were interviewed after the performance only. People were interviewed as they entered and exited the theater venue. To maintain anonymity of participation, respondents were given a number at the time of their first interview; pre- and postperformance interviews were linked by numbers.

Results of the evaluation revealed that after viewing the show participants had improved overall knowledge of HIV/AIDS and specifically of transmission modes; they expressed greater concern about AIDS and were more likely to believe that people could get AIDS from someone who looked healthy, people with AIDS would die from the disease, and AIDS could be prevented.

Little has been published in the literature about strategies for evaluating AIDS-related theater performances and puppet shows. From the perspective of evaluation, the first issue is to determine what outcomes can be expected to change and over what period of time. Evaluation of theater and puppetry performances is challenging because of difficulties with sampling, audience accessibility, people leaving the performance early, and maintaining audience anonymity. The use of a "postintervention-only" group in addition to a preintervention–postintervention group permits disentanglement of intervention versus interview reactivity effects. Process measures, including strengths and weaknesses perceived both by the audience and actors/actresses, can also be used to document the intervention.

While several strategies can be used to measure immediate effects of theatrical intervention, assessment of longer-term outcomes is difficult because of the need for audience anonymity and difficulty in getting the audience to complete a follow-up questionnaire by mail. A pretest–posttest design can be employed to assess knowledge, attitude and intent change by exposing one group (the experimental group) to the theater experience and using another group that has not been exposed to the theater as a control. Both groups are then tested 3 or 6 months after the theater performance to assess behavioral change and stability of cognitive and attitudinal changes. A primary obstacle in executing this design is the success in getting control group members to return for the follow-up assessment. One approach to enhance the return rate of this group is to offer the theater performance to members immediately following their completion of the follow-up questionnaire. This is referred to as a wait-list control group, as described in Chapter 5.

Videos.   Videos are one of the most popular forms of media used by CBOs to educate clients and service providers about HIV. They are particularly appealing to use in hospital and STD clinics and schools because of their captive waiting room audiences. Unfortunately, there is a dearth of published data on their effectiveness as an HIV prevention strategy.

A number of studies (Schoonover, Bassuk, Smith, & Gaskill, 1983; Solomon & De Jong, 1986; Gagliano, 1988; Edgar, Hammond, & Freimuth, 1989; Mushkin & Stevens, 1990) have identified crucial features of a video in bringing about knowledge, attitude, and behavioral change:

- Soap opera style story line that builds tension.
- Role modeling of desired behaviors by actors and actresses with similar socio-demographic characteristics as the target audience.
- Messages based on the target audience's vernacular language.
- Emotional appeal.

Videos may be used as the sole intervention strategy or in conjunction with other modalities. Effectiveness of videos relative to other types of interventions, such as discussion, has been assessed. Often, video interventions are delivered in a single session. For example, a videotape intervention, *The Subject Is AIDS*, was compared to two other educational approaches: (1) written informational materials, and (2) a nurse educator encounter, with a randomized controlled design among 217 women enrolled in the Women, Infants, and Children (WIC) program (Ashworth, DuRant, Gaillard, & Rountree, 1994). The interventions lasted between 15 to 18 minutes.

Prior to randomization, all women completed a pretest focusing on AIDS knowledge, concern about personal risk, and risk behaviors. Immediately following the intervention, participants completed a posttest questionnaire designed to measure short-term knowledge gain and attitudinal changes. A second posttest assessment was administered 2 months later, which was conducted to determine retention of knowledge and maintenance of attitudinal and behavioral change. Results indicated that while the video and nurse education groups showed immediate increases in AIDS knowledge postintervention compared to the information only control group, this increase was not retained at the 2-month follow-up assessment. In terms of risk-taking behavior, the videotape group had a significant decrease immediately following the intervention, but increased this behavior at the 2-month follow-up. The researchers suggest that the video may have been more effective in the short-run because participants were swept up by the emotional intensity of the message.

AIDS Is about Secrets, a 37-minute video developed by the HIV Center for Clinical and Behavioral Studies at the New York State Psychiatric Institute (1989) in collaboration with members of African-American and Latino communities in New York City, traces the stories of four women struggling with their susceptibility to and possible infection with HIV. To evaluate the video, a pretest–posttest design was used (Goldfarb, Ehrhardt, Hoffman, Zawadski, & Elkin, 1993). Women were recruited from drug treatment and community centers to participate in a 2-hour focus group to view the video and discuss it following the viewing. A $20 financial incentive was provided. Eight focus groups were convened, with a total of 57 participants. Program impact was assessed by whether the intervention:

- Increased participants' perceptions of personal risk for HIV infection.
- Increased participants' self-efficacy around protecting oneself from HIV.
- Changed participants' attitudes and intended behaviors regarding condom use.
- Changed participants' attitudes and behaviors regarding sexual communication.
- Identified characteristics of the video that may account for its effectiveness or ineffectiveness.

Prior to viewing the video, participants completed a pretest assessing demographics, perceptions of personal risk for HIV, self-efficacy regarding HIV prevention, as well as attitudes and behaviors regarding condom use and sexual communication. The posttest questionnaire tapped the same domains as the pretest, except for behavior items, which were reworded to reflect intended rather than actual behaviors.

Impact evaluation examined changes in the targeted outcomes. Qualitative analysis was used to develop and code themes emerging from the focus group discussions. Quantitative analyses revealed that the women were more likely to say that long-term sexual partners often kept secrets about drug use from others and were less likely to say that they would know whether or not their partners were engaging in risky behavior. In other words, the women reported an increase in healthy skepticism about their partner's professed behavior that might put them at risk. Also, a significant positive change was noted in intention to get their partner to use condoms consistently. The qualitative analyses corroborated the quantitative findings and showed additional information that could not be gleaned from the quantitative assessment.

A content analysis of the focus group discussions examined the following dimensions:

- Credibility of the characters and situations
- Identification with the characters
- Reactions to language
- Reactions to production style

This component of the evaluation revealed that women liked the realism of the video and, in particular, could identify with the character showing inner fortitude.

Because there was no follow-up beyond the immediate postvideo assessment, the long-term effects of the video on the audience are unknown. Thus, repeated postintervention assessments should be considered. Also, without a control group, any changes in outcomes could not be attributed to the video.

Home Risk-Reduction Parties. These are a form of peer education. In this single-event intervention, peer/health educators provide a prevention message, e.g., safer sex or safer drug use, to members of his or her community.

A one-time 3½-hour peer-led discussion group for a "Stop AIDS" program targeted to sexual risk reduction among self-identified gay and bisexual men in Orange County, California, was evaluated with a pre- and posttest design in which participants completed a self-administered AIDS prevention test before and after the discussion group (Miller, Booraem, Flowers, & Iversen, 1990). The questionnaire assessed HIV-related knowledge, attitudes, and commitment to behavior change. Subjects were recruited from places where gay men were known to congregate. The discussion groups consisted of 4 to 15 participants and were conducted in private homes. As there were no normative data, half of the participants completed the tests in the reverse order, that is, the posttest version of the questionnaire was completed prior to the group discussion and the pretest version after the group discussion. While study findings indicated significant changes in the knowledge, attitude, and behavioral intentions domains, knowledge was not correlated with attitude change and only minimally correlated with behavioral intentions from pretest to posttest. The two major shortcomings of this evaluation approach were the lack of a comparison group and assessment of longer-term intervention effects, such as actual behavioral change.

Multisession Interventions

Workshops. A multisessioned health education program is where the same group of respondents participate in all sessions. Examples of these types of interventions include skills-building and problem-solving workshops and training programs.

Skills-Building/Problem-Solving Workshops. Many community-based and health care organizations conduct one-time workshops to educate their staff and clientele about HIV infection, transmission, and prevention methods. The focus of these workshops is often didactic, with a lecture and/or presentation followed by question-and-answer period. Evaluation can be built into the workshop design and plan. Since it may only be possible to ask participants questions while they are attending the workshop, such evaluation will be limited to assessing the impact of the workshop on participants' knowledge and attitudes. Behavior cannot be expected to change immediately after the workshop, and therefore should not be assessed unless a follow-up survey will be administered several months after the workshop. Within the knowledge domain, changes in levels of awareness, transmission methods, and symptoms of HIV can be assessed. Within the attitudinal domain, changes in attitudes about casual contact with people with AIDS, sexual intercourse with an HIV-infected person, homosexuality, substance abuse, the efficacy of medical treatment, childbearing among HIV-infected women, condom use, HIV testing, and partner referral can be explored as they relate to workshop content. Also, changes in levels of self-confidence, e.g., ability to seek confidential HIV testing if concerned about exposure, and in the ability to transmit HIV knowledge to others can be assessed (Bell *et al.*, 1990). Example 9.5 illustrates an HIV/AIDS skills-building workshop among clients in drug treatment.

When workshop attendees participate anonymously, follow-up assessment is problematic. A mail follow-up cannot be done, and participants cannot be telephoned. There are several viable options, however. Participants can be given a card at the workshop with an appointment to return to complete the questionnaire. On the actual return date, after completion of the questionnaire, an educational and social event in which refreshments are served could be held. A second method entails distributing follow-up questionnaires with addressed, stamped envelopes at the workshop and asking participants to complete the questionnaire at the specified assessment period and then mail the questionnaires or drop them in a designated box at the sponsoring CBO's office. In any event, if the design calls for matching across points in time, it is necessary to encode a unique identification number that will identify the protocol but maintain the anonymity of the participant.

Example 9.5.   Project HOPE, New York City

Intervention Description

Project HOPE (Health Options through Preventive Education) was an HIV risk-reduction program for men and women in two drug treatment programs in New York City. The single-gender, six-session workshops were designed to reduce the incidence of unintended pregnancy and HIV transmission. Intervention content included didactic sessions, role play, and vignettes.

Evaluation Design

Data were collected using a semistructured interview tool. Participants were interviewed prior to participation and 6 and 12 months postintervention.

Sample

Five hundred nineteen African-American and Latino men and women completed the pretest. Of the 284 women who pretested, 147 completed the 6-month follow-up and 88 completed the 12-month follow-up. Of the 235 men who completed baseline, 104 and 59 completed 6- and 12-month assessments, respectively.

Results

Condom use increased significantly from baseline to 6-month follow-up for both men ($P < 0.001$) and women ($P < 0.02$), as did sexual self-efficacy ($P < 0.005$ and $P = 0.02$, respectively). Gains in condom use and sexual self-efficacy were maintained from the 6- to 12-month follow-up period.

(SOURCE: Mantell, Ramos, Karp, & Roman, 1995b.)

Counselor Training. Frequently, health educators will be asked to evaluate whether the quality of AIDS training given to service providers has been effective. Training can be in the form of multisession workshops using a variety of teaching techniques, such as cognitive–behavioral skills training and videotapes. This training may have different goals, e.g., improving providers' knowledge about HIV, their counseling skills, or ability to manage HIV patients. Training can be evaluated using one or a variety of methods, e.g., didactic, didactic role play, and modeling. Training effectiveness needs to be assessed in terms of initial effects as well as longer-term consequences. Are the gains in knowledge or skills that have been achieved immediately following the training maintained over time?

Both process and impact measures can be used to evaluate training. Process measures address problems encountered in the training and trainers' performance, while impact measures assess changes in trainees' knowledge, attitudes, and behaviors, such as anxiety about working with HIV-infected individuals, death anxiety, homophobia, or client satisfaction with the counseling session.

For longer-term evaluation, you may want to determine whether counselors have improved their empathy skills. Empathy would be difficult to determine immediately after training. An evaluator also must determine how improvement in this skill can best be measured. One technique is to use vignettes to assess this construct indirectly. Do the counselors have the capacity to empathize with clients' situations? Assessment can be conducted on a one-to-one basis or with a group of individuals.

A third area for evaluation relates to client outcomes. Assessing client outcomes, however, is problematic in that assessment of the counselors' clients would be required. The number of clients who were counseled can be documented as a process measure. In addition, the evaluator may want to compare the effectiveness of a peer educator/counselor indigenous to the target population versus a health care professional on client outcomes. This can be achieved with the use of a quasi-experimental design.

Example 9.6 illustrates one strategy used to evaluate a training workshop on AIDS counseling. Findings from the evaluation underscore the importance of knowing the audience and targeting the training accordingly. The evaluation included both process and impact measures; whether the training improved the health professionals' skills and ultimately their clients' risk reduction is unknown.

Community-Level Interventions

In these types of interventions, the overall goal is to have an impact on the community as a whole. Here, a target strategy is designed to foster community change as a function of the intervention. Examples of these types of intervention modalities include outreach, ethnographic intervention, small media, and mass media.

Outreach

Outreach is a popular HIV prevention strategy, particularly with populations that researchers have found difficult to reach, such as IDUs, sex workers, the homeless, and runaway youth. This has stimulated a generation of innovative programs that characteristically take the prevention program to the community—the streets and other natural venues—and use peers as messengers of HIV prevention. These programs include syringe exchange, HIV screening in hotel rooms or mobile vans, education and distribution of condoms and other prevention materials to youth, and dissemination of small media materials to housing project residents. Attempts to evaluate these programs have been minimal. Example 9.7 describes one outreach program that had an evaluation component.

Syringe Exchange Programs. Because of the decidedly controversial though promising nature of syringe exchange programs, it is essential that they be properly and effectively evaluated. By distributing new, free sterile syringes, such programs are believed to reduce the sharing of dirty needles, and thus stem the spread of HIV infection. Critics of such programs argue that they encourage drug injection and increase the number of IDUs. To date, studies have not shown that syringe exchange increases drug use or injection (Van den Hoek, Van Haastrecht, & Coutinho, 1989; Buning, Van Brussel,

---

Example 9.6. The National AIDS Counselling
Training Unit, United Kingdom

Intervention Description

The National AIDS Counselling Training Unit in London evaluated a series of small-group workshops to train health care workers in a range of counseling skills. Training began in 1985 and was conducted on weekends.

Evaluation Strategy

A random sample of 100 consecutive health care workers drawn at the end of 1987 was assessed immediately prior to the workshop, immediately after the training, and by mail 6 months after completing their workshop to determine long-term impact of the counseling training. The mail return rate was greater than 75%. The evaluation sought to understand the needs of participants, difficulties and obstacles they encountered, and the effectiveness of the workshops in addressing these needs. Assessment covered the following areas:

- AIDS anxiety
- Patterns of contact with people with HIV infection, need for different kinds of AIDS information, counseling skills, and psychological techniques to manage patients
- Course content
- Perceptions of the extent to which individuals could influence services
- Usefulness of workshop
- Appraisal of stress as a result of working in the field of AIDS

Results

The workshops reduced anxiety about contact with and counseling people with HIV/AIDS at both the immediate and 6-month follow-up. In general, participants did not report their work to be stressful. There were no differences in participants' patterns of contact with people with HIV/AIDS at 6-month follow-up. The need for counseling skills, psychological management, basic information about AIDS, and pre- and posttest counseling was rated high by participants. The majority were interested in follow-up courses and small in-depth workshops were the preferred method.

(SOURCE: Sherr & McCreaner, 1989.)

& Van Santen, 1988; Guydish *et al.*, 1993; Kaplan & Heimer, 1995). Rather, results show that such programs decrease needle sharing among IDUs.

Relevant indicators of program success would be any behaviors that reduce HIV transmission. Over the past several years, systematic evaluation of syringe exchange programs has increased. As Stimson (1989) points out in his review of these programs,

---

Example 9.7. The Central London Action in Street Health (CLASH)

Intervention Description

Health education outreach and referrals to health and social services for sex workers and IDUs were implemented. Outreach was undertaken in the streets, subway stations, pubs, cafes, syringe exchanges, prisons, and youth clubs.

Evaluation Strategy

A combination of qualitative and quantitative techniques were used. Process-oriented evaluation focused on the extent to which program objectives were met, including nature and extent of involvement in program, project feasibility and effectiveness of management structure and functioning, problems with management, perceived feasibility and effectiveness of outreach activities, and collaboration between outreach staff and community organizations. Qualitative methods included documentation of project history and start-up, observations of outreach team, participant observation in streets (once a week for 18 months), in-depth interviews with outreach workers, staff of community agencies, and other key informants. Some intermediate outcome evaluation was also conducted. Findings related to project performance and intermediate outcome measures were fed back to outreach workers and managers and HIV service coordinators.

(SOURCE: Rhodes & Holland, 1992.)

---

evaluation research efforts have been impeded by the need for anonymous participation due to the illegal nature of injecting drugs and the distribution of syringes without a prescription.

Evaluation has consisted primarily of surveys of users' self-reported changes in knowledge, attitudes, and behaviors and the return rate of syringes. As with self-reports of sexual behavior, the frequency of the behavior (needle sharing) cannot be monitored; in addition, social desirability bias effects associated with self-reported behavior could result in low frequency of self-reported needle-sharing behavior. Ultimately, however, the long-term criterion of syringe exchange program success is a reduction in new HIV infections among the IDU population. Decreased incidence of HIV infections has not yet been definitively linked with syringe exchange interventions.

Few evaluation plans for interventions in the early years of the HIV epidemic included a control or comparison group of nonparticipants. The use of a control or comparison group will help the researcher to determine whether changes in participants' knowledge, attitudes or behaviors are attributed to attending the syringe exchange program or to other factors, such as media campaigns or increased TV coverage (Donoghoe, Stimson, Dolan, & Alldritt, 1989b). Other methodological flaws that have affected program evaluation efforts are inadequate follow-up, sampling bias, small sample size, and subject attrition (Stimson, 1989).

HIV seroprevalence of "hidden" populations is difficult to estimate because the denominator is frequently unknown. This problem has already been demonstrated with the homeless and untreated IDUs. One method is a capture–recapture approach used by McKeganey, Barnard, Bloor, and Leyland (1990) to study street prostitutes in which new field contacts are distinguished from repeat field contacts and injectors from noninjectors. Sterile injecting equipment was distributed and provided another measure of frequency of injection besides self-reported drug use. Monitoring the rate of return of syringes, which are frequently marked with color bands or tracking numbers for study purposes, provides an unobtrusive method of evaluation that is not dependent on self-report (Guydish *et al.*, 1991). The capture–recapture approach also permits assessment of the extent to which different distribution sites reach diverse IDU populations.

Designed to reduce and eliminate the sharing of needles and "works" (sharing of syringes, cookers, and needles) among IDUs, the syringe exchange at St. Mary's Hospital in London used a number of indicators to evaluate program success, including a survey of clients' perceptions of the service, their drug use and sexual behaviors, and the number of times they took advantage of those services provided (Mulleady *et al.*, 1988).

Other evaluation parameters for syringe exchange are:

- Total number of clients.
- Number of new clients receiving service.
- Total number of client visits.
- Frequency of recent injecting and sharing.
- Length of time syringes have circulated before being returned.
- Number of condoms distributed.
- Mean number of noninjecting sexual partners. While this is not a measure of risk reduction for the injector, the risk of HIV infection increases for the noninjecting partner who is a sex partner of an IDU (Donoghoe, Stimson, & Dolan, 1989a).
- Number of clients who continue the practice of high-risk sexual behaviors.
- Clients' increased use of condoms.
- Number of clients who continue drug use, but cease injecting.
- Number of clients who inject but stop sharing equipment..
- Abstinence from drug use.
- Changes in clients' HIV-related knowledge and attitudes.
- Number of clients referred for drug treatment.

Syringe exchange tracking and testing are integral to the evaluation of New Haven's needle exchange program (Kaplan, 1991). In addition to outcomes already noted, the person who receives the syringe as well as the person who returns the syringe are monitored. Returned syringes are tested to determine whether they contain infected blood. This is often difficult because the syringe may contain only a small amount of blood for HIV testing. Tracking is possible because participants are given fictitious names.

Another evaluation strategy used to determine whether the presence of a syringe exchange program increases injecting drug use has been to investigate all drug treatment admissions in a community prior to and following the implementation a syringe exchange program, as described in Example 9.8. As these researchers note, because data on

---

Example 9.8. Evaluation Strategy for a Syringe
Exchange Program, San Francisco, California

Two years prior to implementation of their needle exchange program, admission data to all county-funded drug treatment facilities in San Francisco were compared to comparable data 2 years following its implementation. Analyses of all admissions, regardless of the number of discrete patients, provided an indicator of community-level effects. Multiple means of assessment were employed. First, based on all admissions, the proportion reporting injection drug use over four 1-year consecutive periods was used to determine whether injection drug use had increased. Second, among those who reported injection drug use, the frequency of injection in the previous 30 days between the four time periods was assessed. Third, in the one methadone detoxification clinic that reported needle-sharing data over the entire study period, self-reported needle-sharing practices, e.g., number of needle-sharing partners, number of needle-sharing occasions in the 30 days preceding treatment, were documented. Fourth, to evaluate whether the program encouraged noninjecting drug users to begin injecting, retrospective cohorts of individuals who had repeated drug treatment-related admissions were compared before and after the introduction of the syringe exchange program. Finally, census tract data were used to compare two high-drug use neighborhoods with exchange sites to two high-drug use neighborhoods without the exchange program. In particular, the proportion of those entering treatment, and among the IDUs the age at first injection and current frequency of injection, in the exchange and nonexchange communities were compared.

(SOURCE: Guydish *et al.*, 1993.)

---

the needle exchange status of the sample were not collected, the behavior of IDUs participating in the exchange with those who did not participate could not be compared. The generalizability of findings to drug users not enrolled in drug treatment cannot be ascertained. As with the other studies reported above, bias due to self-reporting and recall problems could affect the validity of findings. Also, history effects due to changes in San Francisco's drug treatment system, e.g., increased number of treatment slots and specialized programs targeted to women and crack cocaine users, can affect conclusions about program effects.

Ethnographic Intervention

As noted in Chapter 7, ethnographic methods may include intervention. Ethnographic intervention refers to the provision of services and the active participation of the group or community under prolonged study in addition to traditional data collection methods. In the area of HIV/AIDS prevention, Wiebel (1988) developed an ethnographic intervention approach for drug users in Chicago. Intervention was designed to: (1) identify and access target populations with the use of indigenous fieldworkers; these fieldworkers serve as HIV prevention advocates, delivering services at sites where IDUs congregate; (2) increase a group's or community's understanding of HIV—their knowledge, attitudes, and behaviors; (3) encourage individuals to appraise realistically their personal risk for HIV infection and evaluate the adoption of viable options to high-risk behaviors; (4) reinforce HIV risk-reduction practices through repeated exposure in multiple contexts; and (5) extend the impact of the ethnographic intervention by fostering norms for "prevention advocacy" in IDUs' social networks. Ethnographic intervention with drug users can also be used to monitor trends in drug practices over time and their consequences for HIV transmission (Koester, 1994).

Employing indigenous workers who have an in-depth understanding of the drug lifestyle (and therefore are able to gain the trust of the drug-using population) as HIV prevention advocates is an important factor in community acceptance of the intervention. To reduce the risk of HIV infection and limit further transmission among drug users and their sexual partners, other intervention strategies, including distribution of condoms, bleach, and educational materials, informal and semistructured interviews with key informants and community leaders, and direct observation of events and physical environments, can be employed.

Ethnographic intervention also has been frequently aimed at sex workers "on the stroll" to educate them about safer sex and drug-injecting practices. Education is provided through one-to-one intervention on the street, as well as through workshops and drop-in support groups in community storefront settings. Free bleach, condoms, and educational materials are distributed. Evaluation indicators for this type of intervention include: (1) the number of safer sex and bleach kits distributed; (2) changes in distribution over time; (3) increase in demand for the kits; and (4) changes in knowledge, attitudes, and beliefs as determined by periodic formal interviews with small groups of women.

Based on the various sources of ethnographic data collected and noted above, the evaluator will have to determine the amount of change necessary to consider the outreach program a success. As with quantitative data collection methods, program success criteria should be defined at the outset, rather than after the data are collected.

Ethnographic field workers systematically record in diaries or logs their impressions of observations and interactions with the population in various sites of the target community. These field note data are subsequently analyzed and interpreted. One example of elements of systematic data collection is the structured observation form used in Macquarie University's (Australia) Bisexually Active Men's Outreach Project (Davis, Klemmer, & Dowsett, 1991), presented in Table 9.9. A fieldworker kept a diary of his impressions from participant observation and interactions with bisexually active men on "beats" or cruising areas. This observation provided the project staff with descriptions of the sex scene and the individuals who cruised, and thus some indication of the HIV-related sexual risk behaviors among this population of "cruisers."

Data from field notes become the basis for planning and prioritizing future outreach activities and other types of interventions. The use of ethnographic intervention, in which unstructured interviews and HIV testing were employed to document injecting drug practices, for planning and implementing appropriate intervention is described in Example 9.9.

Another illustration of the use of ethnographic intervention to provide HIV/AIDS

Table 9.9. Selected Variables to Consider in Observing a "Beat"[a]

Description of the "beat"
  Physical layout of the setting
  Demographic profile of users
  How the beat works
Observations of the men
  What happened?
  Describe the educational opportunities
  How can education be provided within the context of limited contact with target population?
Interactions with bisexually active men
  How do bisexually active men conduct their daily lives?
  What do they do on the beat? Do they talk with others on the beat?
Sexuality
  What words are used?
  What are they reticent to talk about?
  How defensive are they in talking about their sexual lifestyle?
Sexual practices
  How often do they use the beats? What kind of sex do they like to have?
  What do they do for sex and thrills?
  How do they negotiate sex? How do they talk about sex with their partner? Their wives?
  What are the patterns of nonverbal interaction?

[a]From Davis *et al.* (1991) with permission.

Example 9.9. Ethnographic Interview Guide
for Study of Injection Drug Users

In Seattle, ethnographic studies of two communities of IDUs (racially and ethnically diverse heterosexual and homosexual IDUs) were conducted to determine their extent of risk for HIV infection and the specific modes of transmission. A sample of IDUs was recruited through a modified chain-referral technique in which those IDUs interviewed recommended other IDUs to be contacted about study participation. HIV testing was offered. The data were used to plan and develop appropriate interventions that were acceptable to the target population. Themes for the ethnographic interview guide to document injecting drug use and sharing of "works" were:

- Beliefs about needle use
- Where and how needles are obtained
- Who obtains the needles
- The cost of the needles
- The context in which the needles are shared or not shared
- Whether sharing occurs more often in some situations than others
- Who shares needles
- Whether and how often sharing occurs across lines of race, social class, and sexual orientation

(Source: Kleyn *et al.*, 1988.)

prevention is the in-depth study of migrant farm workers in Michigan (Bletzer, 1995). This method was particularly fitting because of the lack of information about their sexual risk behaviors, rates of HIV infection, and how to introduce health-related materials to this population.

Implementation of the intervention to increase migrant workers' understanding of HIV risk behaviors and data collection were concurrent. Intervention activities included presentation of a video. Data collection strategies consisted of field notes on language use, behavioral responses to the video, interactions between the educator and group as well as among participants, and interviews with male and female adults and adolescents and couples. A content analysis (i.e., an analysis of narrative text), used to catalogue themes and reduce the data, was performed on the field notes of responses to the video showings and a discourse or conversation analysis of the recorded interactions.

The educator/evaluator's observation of reactions to the video revealed that the scenarios on extramarital sex and sex between men (even if they were married) were the two most frequently noticed segments of the video, as expressed through the migrant workers' display of surprise and laughter. This observation was confirmed by their verbal comments. The content analysis showed that the video scenes pertaining to drug use and needle-cleaning were inappropriate for this population. It also provided insight into gender-role norms regarding extramarital consensual sex between men, marital fidelity, and women's allegiance to their spouses, as well as willingness to talk about AIDS and personal risk behaviors in a formal setting. Thus, data analyses pinpointed areas for future intervention and documented effective strategies of communicating HIV prevention messages.

Small Media

Small media refer to controlled print and audiovisual media with limited distribution. This includes videos, brochures and pamphlets, newsletters, posters, and other print materials.

Videos.   In an intervention and evaluation currently underway, a video, *Rompiendo el Silencio* (Breaking the Silence) (HIV Center for Clinical and Behavioral Studies at the New York State Psychiatric Institute, 1994), is used as part of a larger New York City study on diffusion-of-innovation model to assess the effectiveness of prevention messages based on an AIDS education video. The model focuses on the role of social networks in promoting or impeding safer-sex negotiations and practices among heterosexual Latinas. Two aspects of the video were assessed: (1) its prevention messages, and (2) characteristics of the video (e.g., viewers' identification with characters, relevance to viewers' life).

A pretest–posttest design, with a baseline and two follow-up assessments (following the video viewing and the group discussion, and three months after the baseline) was used (Ortiz-Torres & Ehrhardt, 1995; Ortiz-Torres, Ehrhardt, Van Dommelen, Del Carmen Rivera, & Rivera, 1996). The pretest tapped such domains as perceived social norms, normative beliefs, sexual behavior in the past 3 months, and demographics. The first posttest assessed the prevention messages, the video itself, and changes in normative beliefs, perceived norms, and behavioral intentions. A second posttest assessed changes in women's normative beliefs and protective behaviors, retention of messages from the video, and whether participants diffused HIV prevention messages to others in their social network. Diffusion was operationalized by the average number of network members shown the video by each participant and the total average number of individuals who had seen the video 3 months after the intervention. Extending the window period for follow-up assessment would enable the evaluator to determine whether any changes in normative beliefs and social norms evident at the first or second follow-ups would be maintained.

AIDS Prevention Brochures, Posters, and Other Printed Materials. A major method of disseminating information to communities is the use of brochures. Such pamphlets are typically used in conjunction with other intervention strategies. While brochures do not usually lead to behavioral change, they can increase people's awareness of AIDS as well as reinforce HIV risk-reduction practices. For example, to evaluate AIDS prevention brochures for male and female undergraduate students (D'Augelli & Kennedy, 1989), several dimensions were examined. Seven are listed below:

- Precision of information.
- Suitability for teens and parents.
- Information about how to avoid AIDS.
- Decision-making skills concerning sexual practices and drug use.
- Guidelines for safer sex.
- Frequency of condom discussion.
- Importance of discussing AIDS with sexual partners and for safer sex.

Critical to the effectiveness of the small media campaign is the degree to which it is monitored. Monitoring enables the evaluator to determine the extent to which the planned activities (poster or brochure) are actually being implemented. The evaluator surveys the users of the printed material to determine if the target audience is being reached with the intended message. Techniques such as "on-the-street" interviews or more formal focus groups are commonly used to monitor the effectiveness of a small media campaign.

Thousands of printed HIV educational materials such as posters, brochures, and pamphlets have been developed over the last decade, yet only a small proportion of them have been systematically evaluated. Evaluation is especially important for learning whether materials are relevant to their target audiences. As noted in Chapter 7, focus groups are especially useful in evaluating written materials. Example 9.10 illustrates the use of formative evaluation with a focus group to evaluate an AIDS prevention poster.

Mass Media-Based Interventions

Media-based campaigns have been the primary vehicle for disseminating AIDS information to the general public. Mass media have the advantage of reaching a large audience through such means as television specials (e.g., *An Early Frost*), sitcoms featuring characters who use condoms, talk shows, newscasts, soaps, videos, music,

---

Example 9.10. Formative Evaluation
of an AIDS Education Poster, South Africa

Sample

Literate, black, sexually active urban men and women in Johannesburg, South Africa.

Evaluation Strategy

To evaluate the appropriateness of a cartoon and condom prevention message as a poster, six focus groups homogeneous by gender were conducted. Group members were systematically selected from Johannesburg Health Department STD, family planning, and TB clinics, and City Council domestic workers, security officers, drivers, and clerks. The poster was shown to group members for 60-second time limit; after this viewing, group members were interviewed to determine their understanding of the poster and its prevention message. Time was allotted to allow the group to discuss among themselves their reactions to the poster. The poster was then shown to the group for a second time without a time limit, and the evaluators asked questions about phrases, pictures, and the poster design. The discussion was tape-recorded and handwritten notes were taken. At the end of the group session, the group was able to ask the facilitator questions about the poster's content.

Results

While group members understood the prevention messages (Stick to one partner. Use a condom if you don't know your partner very well), the captioned words of the woman in the poster were vague and ambiguous. Group members did not understand that the main message—AIDS won't just go away; take care—meant that condoms should be used for protection. The strong anticondom sentiment and barriers to condom use among the target audience were also revealed. Barriers included the association of condoms with STDs, mistrust of sexual partners, and inaccessibility in the community. Feedback from the evaluation resulted in modification of the poster—more direct and literal messages, simpler typeface, and explicit information about where to get assistance.

(SOURCE: Evian, Ijsselmuiden, Padayachee, & Hurwitz, 1990.)

---

newspapers, billboards, posters, pamphlets, public service announcements (PSAs), computer bulletin boards, and employee newsletters. Conventional wisdom suggests that a wide range of complementary media communication strategies and prevention messages are needed to reach multiple audiences. Television, in particular, is a powerful tool for promoting health information, generating positive and negative reinforcements for health behavior through the use of role models, and reducing the stigma associated with AIDS (Wallack, 1990).

AIDS health messages may attempt to change knowledge, attitudes, and risk behavior, but there is little evidence that they bring about behavioral change. In the short-run, such campaigns have been shown to increase recognition of risk, but do not necessarily achieve desired behavior change (Flora, Maccoby, & Farquhar, 1989). The latter may require a longer time frame. They are also sometimes disappointing because despite saturating a market, they may be viewed by a relatively small proportion of the intended audience (Edgar *et al.*, 1989). Television and radio PSAs may not be aired as frequently as desired or are aired at hours not watched or listened to by the target population because they depend on donated time.

Factors such as the social environment, personal characteristics and motivations of the audience to reduce their risk, and the content of the messages themselves may affect the degree to which a campaign is proved to be effective. Other factors that may affect program success include: (1) the timing of the data collection (e.g., the longer the time period between pre- and posttest assessment and the more information presented, the greater the increases in AIDS knowledge); (2) the date of the public information campaign (e.g., evaluation of campaigns conducted after intensive media intervention may not show significant changes due to ceiling or saturation effects compared to campaigns conducted before extensive media involvement); and (3) uncontrolled extraneous factors may cloud true effects.

Public service announcements are one of the primary channels of communicating AIDS messages to the public. Cardinal features of PSAs are narrow program objectives disseminated over a defined period of time and messages directed to modify or reinforce audience knowledge and attitudes. These campaigns may aim to reach a national audience or specific groups defined by geographic region, demographic characteristics, or their practice of HIV risk behaviors. Emotional messages have been found to stimulate viewers to seek further information about AIDS more so than rational messages and to be more likely to be remembered by people for whom AIDS is not personally relevant, i.e., those who are not at risk for HIV (Flora & Maibach, 1990). Evaluation of media campaigns can tell us how effective mass media is in transferring AIDS information to the general population, populations at risk for HIV, service providers, and clinicians.

Process evaluation measures of media campaigns include:

- Venue for information dissemination (churches, clinics, community, CBOs).
- Characteristics of the audience reached.
- Number of times target audience was exposed to the message.
- Reactions of audience to prevention message.
- Amount of money and personnel resources required to achieve desired outcome.
- Monitoring the number of information requests made through calls to hotlines.

Focus groups or interviews with members of the target group are often a primary means for testing the copy of a campaign message. Repeated cross-sectional surveys are frequently used to monitor the effects of a campaign. Samples of the general population may be used to assess recall, understanding, persuasion, and self-reported behavioral change (Coyle *et al.*, 1991). To control for confounding by extraneous factors, surveys should also be conducted in control communities that are not exposed to the campaign.

A case study of a mass media campaign is described below.

Case Study: America Responds to AIDS (ARTA)

Intervention Description. A multimedia, multiphase campaign was initiated in 1987 by the Centers for Disease Control to heighten public awareness and understanding of HIV/AIDS and increase public sensitivity to the plight of people with HIV (US Centers for Disease Control, 1991a). Radio and television PSAs (in 1987) and the mailing of a brochure about AIDS to every US household (in mid-1988) were used to reach the general public. In addition, targeted PSA campaigns were directed to women at risk for AIDS and sexually active adults with multiple partners (in 1988) and parents and youth (in 1989). Printed PSAs, brochures, and posters were displayed in mass transit systems (e.g., on buses, subways, and in taxis), in doctors' offices, pharmacies, and libraries.

Evaluation Strategy. To evaluate the short-term efficacy of two ARTA television PSAs, a field study was conducted in two sites: Springfield, Illinois, and Memphis, Tennessee (Siska, Jason, Murdoch, Shan Yang, & Donovan, 1992). The two PSAs were randomly assigned to these sites. The evaluation sought to answer four questions: (1) Did either PSA increase awareness of AIDS as an important national issue? (2) Did people remember the PSA? (3) Was one PSA more effective than the other in increasing public awareness of AIDS or recall of the PSA? (4) Did either PSA produce negative effects?

One week prior to the study, a random-digit dialing survey of 4181 eligible households was conducted; of these households, 46% declined study participation, and 8% did not receive the TV channels on which the PSAs were to be aired. The 46% ($n = 1931$) who agreed to participate were then randomly assigned to the experimental group that was to view the PSA or to the unexposed control group. However, only 907 (47%) actually completed the follow-up questionnaire. Participants were asked to watch one of two local late news programs and then asked to list "the most important health and national issues facing our county today." In each city, one station agreed not to air any AIDS PSAs. After the PSAs were aired, follow-up telephone interviews were conducted.

Results. There were higher recall rates in the experimental groups in both cities compared to the controls, although the rate was higher in Tennessee than Illinois. At both sites, the proportion of participants who mentioned AIDS as an important issue increased from recruitment to follow-up for the experimental (from 20.8 to 32.2% in Memphis, and 9.9 to 16.6% in Springfield) but not the control groups. Neither PSA was found to produce negative effects. Limitations of this evaluation included unexpected changes in the scheduling of the PSAs due to the National Basketball Association playoffs and a low participation rate. Whether these increases in awareness and ability to recall the PSAs were maintained over time is unknown.

Media-based interventions can also be directed toward specific groups rather than the entire public. At times, these communities are easily identified. Residents in home-less shelters, clients of drug-free therapeutic communities, and the tenants of a particular housing project are all examples of "closed communities." By this it is meant that they are defined by their membership in a clearly delineated location. Other communities are less easily defined. The next set of examples will demonstrate how these smaller communities within the population can be reached through an intervention.

As described in Example 9.11, college-aged students were the primary target population. Caron, Davis, Wynn, and Roberts (1992, p. 27) concluded that

Target Population

College students.

Evaluation Strategy

Taking advantage of the *America Responds to AIDS* campaign, data were collected from 125 students, mainly freshmen and sophomores enrolled in a social psychology class. The purpose was to evaluate the impact of the campaign on changes in knowledge, attitudes, and practices. Students were interviewed in March 1987, preceding the CDC campaign by several months. A second survey was conducted with a comparable sample of 112 students in September 1988, several months after the mailing of the campaign's brochure to all households in the United States. Questions consisted of: (1) thoughts about AIDS: how students learned about the disease, their knowledge of AIDS; (2) perceived risk: worrying about getting AIDS, about friends worrying, and whether anyone they knew had social, nonsexual contact with HIV-infected individuals, exposure to HIV, considered being tested; (3) beliefs about whether AIDS has had an effect on students' dating behavior and effect on social/bar scene; (4) policy issues concerning condoms, testing, and being HIV-infected; and (5) belief that condoms help prevent the spread of AIDS, location where condoms should be available, and advertising of condoms, opinions about mandatory testing.

Results

In the 1988 sample, personal concern and social concerns were predominant. The majority of both groups first learned about AIDS through the media, but fewer mentioned the media in 1988 (90% in 1987 and 71% in 1988). Significantly more of the 1987 group (24%) compared to 1988 group (10%) reported being prompted to think about it or learning about it through family and friends. Among the two thirds of the 1987 sample who mentioned HIV transmission, 55% gave at least one accurate fact compared to 24% of those who mentioned transmission (55%) in the 1988 group. Of those who reported when they were first concerned, significantly more of the 1988 group (72%) had been concerned for more than a year compared to 57% of the 1987 group. Awareness that AIDS affected everyone increased. In 1988, fewer reported that it was homosexuals who were at risk (4%) compared to 14% in 1987. While there was no difference in the proportion who were personally worried about contracting AIDS in the two samples, a gender effect was apparent. Men reported greater concern than women (75% of the men and 49% of the women in 1987; in 1988, 63% of the men and 44% of the women). More of the 1988 than the 1987 sample indicated that they considered being tested (26% vs. 14%). Regarding dating and sexual behavior, nearly half of the 1987 sample mentioned that AIDS already had an effect, while in 1988, more than three quarters reported this. In 1987, 71% believed in mandatory testing at least for some people, while only 56% felt this way in 1988.

(SOURCE: Caron *et al.*, 1992.)

> ... much of the information about AIDS transmitted through the media and through such means
> as the *America Responds to AIDS* campaign has not reached, or at least has not been inter-
> nalized, by many of these young people. Their knowledge tends to be superficial, and the link
> between that knowledge and their own behavior is often not made.

The strategy used in this example represents a more indirect way in which to evaluate the ARTA campaign. The students were not asked specific questions about the campaign—whether they saw it and their reactions. Therefore, the direct impact of the campaign cannot be assessed with this strategy. Rather, this illustrates the diffusion effects of the ARTA campaign among the college community and should be interpreted as such.

College-aged students are a relatively easy community to define and reach for survey. However, the communities hardest hit by the epidemic are also the hardest to reach. Gay and bisexual men, IDUs, and people with AIDS are often hidden in the general population, making them difficult to identify and hence to reach. Below is a case study that examines the process necessary to mount a community-level HIV prevention campaign targeted to gay and bisexual men in New York City.

Case Study: Condom Use Subway Campaign for Gay/Bisexual Men. GMHC's subway campaign for gay men provides an excellent case study of the processes involved in the development and evaluation of population-specific HIV prevention messages (Manalansan, 1992a,b). To develop a subway campaign for New York City gay men, a three-phase campaign was initiated.

In the first phase, a 10-minute telephone survey was completed with 26 service providers in four boroughs (all except Staten Island, which does not have subways) to provide an overview of problems faced by gay men with respect to HIV prevention. Survey data were used as the basis for the development of a campaign strategy. The questionnaire assessed service providers' degree of familiarity about gay men in their geographic service areas: different groups that comprised the gay population in their area, perceptions of the barriers faced by gay men in practicing safer sex, places where gay men go for various reasons (e.g., recreation, sex, health care), and knowledge of strategic areas where safer sex prevention messages could be placed and of effective media for disseminating the messages.

Survey data revealed the need to take into account the ethnolinguistic, socio-economic, generational, and cultural diversity of men who have sex with men in these communities. The importance of reaching young gay men and gay men of color was stressed by respondents. A number of barriers to safer sex were identified: (1) lack of openness about sexual orientation (e.g., cultural attitudes about homosexuality prevent many Latino men from identifying as gay); (2) inaccessibility to education and health services due to poverty and homelessness; and (3) substance use.

Strategic areas in the community for placing HIV prevention messages noted were public facilities (e.g., libraries, museums, subway stations, phone booths, fences, bill-boards); CBOs, clinics, and shelters; and health clubs/gyms and gay social and recreational venues (e.g., bars, porn theaters, Gay Cable Network, magazines, newspapers). Subway ads were the preferred choice. Based on survey findings, three potential subway campaign messages were drafted.

In the second phase of the campaign, another telephone survey was conducted to elicit AIDS service providers' opinions regarding the draft messages. Thirty-five providers were asked to rate the following draft messages: (1) We're prepared (a multicultural troop of naked men with Boy Scout neckerchiefs and caps); (2) He's great in bed and always uses condoms (an interracial couple walking on the beach); and (3) If you do this, use this (two men undressing each other, with a picture of a condom superimposed in the lower right corner of the picture). Evaluation criteria were:

- Impact of visual messages.
- Clarity of the message.
- Relevance of the message to the gay community.
- Overall rating.

The first message was perceived to be poor by the majority of providers. Concern about the possibility of litigation from the Boy Scouts was voiced. The second and third messages were evaluated as good and very good overall. These messages were construed as positive (consistent condom use was equated with sexual prowess), explicit, and as representing an array of gay men of color. The image of the interracial couple received a mixed review.

The third phase was designed to assess the target population's reactions to the subway campaign. The image and prevention message promoted reflected a composite of those described above. The ads were placed on 44 subway platforms in the four targeted New York City boroughs. For the purposes of evaluation, six subway stops were randomly selected: two each in Brooklyn and Manhattan and one each in the Bronx and Queens. At each site, interviews were conducted on one weekday at three different time intervals: 7 AM–9 AM, 11 AM–1 PM, and 4 PM–6 PM. Male subway riders were approached as they entered and exited the stations and were asked to participate in the survey. A screening instrument was initially administered to ferret out men under 25 and those who did not self-identify as gay or bisexual. The screening instrument also asked about respondents' race/ethnicity and education. The item content of questions asked of those men who met the eligibility criteria is shown in Table 9.10.

Of the 630 male subway riders approached, 499 (79%) refused to participate. Of the 131 men who were screened, only 27 (21%) met the eligibility criteria. All of these 27 men identified as gay. The mean age was 33 years (range from 26 to 52); the majority were Caucasian ($n = 22$). The majority reported seeing the subway ad between two to

Table 9.10. Item Content for GMHC Subway Campaign for Gay Men

Place of residence: New York City or other place; borough
Areas where respondent socializes most often
Sources of information about safer sex: GMHC, gay press, other newspapers and magazines, TV, sexual partners, friends, family members, school, printed materials, counselor, doctor, safer-sex workshops, drug treatment center, other
Features of the ad campaign: Number of times campaign seen; English or Spanish version; global affective reaction to the campaign; discussed campaign with others, and if so, with whom; called GMHC Hotline, and if so, kinds of information seeking (basic HIV/AIDS, transmission, safer sex, HIV testing, counseling/support groups); role model (Do the men in the campaign remind you of your friends and/or sexual partners?)

four times, saw the English version only, and liked the positive nature of the message. No one reported calling the GMHC hotline.

This case example demonstrates the use of both qualitative and quantitative assessment in the design and evaluation of the subway campaign intervention and how information from each phase informed the next phase. The community was involved in the design and pretesting of the messages. With the small size and highly self-selected nature of the sample, the effectiveness of the messages in increasing gay men's awareness of the need for HIV prevention cannot be assessed. Bias can also operate with respect to which male subway riders were approached. A protocol must be established prior to data collection to ensure that interviewers' internal biases (e.g., age, race, physical size) do not lead to selecting certain types of men to approach and others to avoid.

As a way of increasing hotline calls, a message could have been placed on the poster: We're interested in your reactions to the campaign, please call GMHC's hotline. Postcards could have been distributed to all men, regardless of sexual orientation, introducing the campaign and telling the viewing audience that you are interested in their reactions to the safer sex subway campaign targeted to gay men. While this approach solicits the opinions of a broader population than the target group, it avoids the problem of asking men to disclose their sexual orientation to a stranger. Both of these approaches, however, still result in a self-selected convenience sample.

As a community, people with AIDS represent a group that would benefit from tertiary prevention programs (i.e., to prevent social and psychological dysfunction and disability in people with AIDS). However, given the climate in which we live, they are also a hidden population. Special care needs to be taken to reach them with the prevention message and at the same time protect their privacy. The following case study illustrates how this was done with a *Pneumocystis carinii* pneumonia (PCP) prophylaxis campaign for people with AIDS in New York City.

Case Study: PCP Prophylaxis Campaign for People with AIDS. In the following case study, the process of evaluating a GMHC media campaign intended to increase awareness of the efficacy of PCP prophylactic treatment and the need for early intervention among HIV-infected men and women is described. Implications for future GMHC media campaigns are discussed (Manalansan, Frederick, Humes, Moraes, & McDaniel, 1993).

A multimedia approach, including a brochure fact sheet, radio announcements, and subway posters, was used to promote the message about the high mortality from PCP and the need for prophylaxis to prevent its onset. The campaign consisted of three phases:

1. Precopy. A 30-minute phone survey of service providers in AIDS agencies, clinics, and hospitals regarding the information and service needs of people with HIV, scope of services, size of client population and number of HIV-infected clients served, and issues and problems of HIV-infected clients.

2. Copy Testing. Face-to-face 25-minute interviews with HIV-infected persons, primarily Latinos and African Americans. Each interviewee was asked to read the poster and brochure and listen to the radio announcement. These three

forms of media were presented in a random order to control for effects due to order of presentation. Participants were also asked to interpret the messages, comment on their cultural sensitivity, and give suggestions. In addition, the New York State AIDS Institute provided feedback. The interview protocol is presented in Table 9.11. The first segment of the campaign implementation took place between September 6, 1993 and October 31, 1993, and included the broadcast of English and Spanish radio announcements (each 325 times) and placement of subway posters on every other subway car. Brochures were mailed to 800 clinics, hospitals, and social service agencies 1 week before the unveiling of the posters. The second segment took place between December 1, 1993 and February 29, 1994, and consisted primarily of the subway posters.

3. Hotline Call Monitoring. Outcome evaluation relied on data from GMHC's hotline about the number of callers requesting information about PCP. This method was selected because the primary campaign objective was to encourage the audience to seek more information about PCP by calling the hotline. Hotline counselors used checklists to categorize callers and their issues. Callers who asked about PCP treatment and prophylaxis asked if they saw or heard the campaign and their reactions to it. Unfortunately, the checklist did not have a separate category for PCP; calls about PCP were noted under the category of "experimental therapies or drugs" or "AIDS information." Thus, it is difficult to assess the impact of this campaign.

Results of the process evaluation revealed communication problems and an inability to meet the demands of Spanish-speaking callers. Other shortcomings identified were a lack of goal consensus among the designers of the campaign, empirical evidence

Table 9.11. Interview Questions re: Subway Poster[a]

What is this poster telling you? (*Probe*: What is the main message(s) communicated by this poster?)

What kinds of people do you think this poster is talking to? (*Probe*: Is the language directed at any particular group of people?)

What do the colors communicate to you? (*Probe*: Do you like the colors? Why or why not?)

Does this poster give you a particular feeling? (*Probe*: Do the words or colors bring up any feelings in you?)

What does PCP mean to you?

Does this poster make you want to do anything? (*Probe*: Would you tell someone you know about the message in the poster? What would you do to obtain more information about AIDS pneumonia?)

Where do you think this poster should be hung up or displayed?

If you saw this poster on the subway, would you look at it? (*Probe*: What would make you look at it? What about the poster would not attract your attention?)

If you had to say there was one thing you learned from this poster, what would it be? (*Probe*: And what would the second thing be?)

What do you find confusing about the poster? (*Probe*: Is the information in the poster clear?)

What was there about the poster that bothered you? (*Probe*: Did you find anything offensive or maybe upsetting?)

How would you change this poster to make it better?

What does it mean to you to have GMHC on the poster?

[a]From Manalansan (1992c), with permission.

about health promotion theories and media campaigns, long-range planning, and training for hotline staff to deal with new procedures.

Evaluation of the phone survey in the precopy phase identified consistent themes: the need for materials that were appropriate for low-literate populations, people of color, and economically disadvantaged women and adolescents and that provided information about opportunistic infections and treatments. The importance of relating treatment to basic needs such as housing and food was also emphasized.

Data from the copy-testing phase indicated that the respondents had a positive reaction to the poster, radio, and brochure and understood the message. After reading or listening to the campaign materials, the majority said they were motivated to call the hotline or talk to a medical professional.

Evaluation of the hotline call monitoring phase revealed that by the end of October 1993, there were no significant increases in the number of English-speaking callers compared to the 12-month period prior to the campaign, and the number of these calls remained the same in both November and December 1993. Similarly, there was no significant increase in the types of issues presented by callers or changes in the demographic characteristics of the callers, content of the calls, or referrals made. In September 1993, the campaign was launched; less than 1% (0.37% or 177/4481) were related to PCP. Of these 97% ($n = 165$) reported seeing or hearing the campaign. One third ($n = 55$) heard only the radio announcement, seven of whom were Spanish-speaking; 104 reported seeing only the poster, of whom two were Spanish-speaking.

A different picture emerged for the Spanish-speaking callers. The number of Spanish-speaking callers increased between 700% to 1000% during September and October 1993 ($n = 165$ and $n = 119$, respectively). By November, when the radio spots were no longer on the air, the number of Spanish-speaking callers dropped to 9, and in December, the number was 20. Most of the callers asked about general HIV/AIDS information, transmission, symptoms, risk reduction, and safer sex rather than PCP prophylaxis and treatment. Thus, these data suggest that radio spots were more successful than the subway ads in reaching a Spanish-speaking audience.

However, there was a number of limitations of this campaign. First, with the method of impact evaluation—monitoring hotline calls—the findings must be interpreted with caution. Because the checklists used to record information about the calls did not have a category for PCP-related issues, and lacked a systematic protocol for hotline counselors to probe for information, the reliability of the findings may be limited. Second, the effects of disseminating the brochure were not evaluated. Third, each form of media should be evaluated separately so that their effects can be disentangled. At least, findings must be limited to the impact of the full campaign. Differential or cumulative effects are unknown given the current intervention. Finally, the need for adequate numbers of Spanish-speaking hotline counselors should have been addressed prior to the campaign.

The ultimate goal of impact and outcome evaluation is to determine the measurable effects of the intervention. Assessing program effects, or "did the program work," is at the crux of the evaluation. The researcher/evaluator needs to determine, a priori, the level of success necessary to deem the intervention effective.

CONCLUSION

As described throughout this chapter, HIV prevention programs exist in many forms. Program developers, educators, and evaluators need to concentrate their efforts on the programs most effective for the communities targeted. All are accountable to their constituencies to deliver accurate and effective prevention messages. Hence, there is a need for process, and impact outcome evaluation of the preventive interventions delivered.

We have tried to illustrate many of the constructs and concepts reviewed in the previous chapters by tying interventions with evaluation strategies. It is essential for AIDS intervention specialists and evaluators to know their target audience and to "market" the intervention in a manner that is culturally sensitive and competent to the communities involved. At the same time, dissemination of intervention and evaluation findings to the target audience, CBOs, and the general public, though often overlooked, is important. Consequently, marketing and dissemination strategies (e.g., mass media, regional conferences, PSAs, or dispatching technical advisors) need to be incorporated into the intervention planning process. Decisions regarding intervention and evaluation level must be congruent to allow for the interpretation of the meaning of results. Finally, as noted in Chapter 5, close attention must be paid to the effect size (a benchmark for interpreting change due to an intervention so that an evaluator has confidence that he or she is not wasting the community's time with a well-intentioned "shot in the dark") and statistical power (a measure of the magnitude and meaning of significant changes in data) of the intervention.

Conclusion

Society must accept two stark facts in order to address HIV/AIDS effectively. First, no country will remain unscathed by the HIV epidemic, based on the increase of the worldwide incidence of the disease. In the United States, in particular, inner cities are faced with the intractable spread of the disease. Second, "success in HIV prevention often requires helping people make and maintain highly consistent behavior changes, often with very little margin for error or lapses—a challenge virtually unprecedented in the behavioral sciences" (Kelly *et al.*, 1993, p. 1024). Unprecedented challenges require unprecedented responses.

The response to ensure a successful preventive intervention is to mount an approach that is collaborative in nature, including the input from all facets of the community and utilizing all available resources. The initial steps toward this goal are part of the development of a program.

PROGRAM DEVELOPMENT: A MULTIDISCIPLINARY APPROACH

Fortunately, we have learned some important lessons from having to address the horror of AIDS. No single discipline holds the answer to the effective prevention of HIV/AIDS transmission. This realization has led to fewer turf wars and more teamwork. The necessity and value of cross-fertilization among various professional disciplines and collaboration between professionals, paraprofessionals, and members of the target community have been realized. Program planners must also work hand-in-hand with members of the community and evaluators to assess not only the efficacy of the program in changing knowledge, beliefs, attitudes, and behaviors, but also the acceptability of such programs in individual communities. No matter how beautifully designed on paper, a program is doomed to failure if the program developers have not tailored the intervention to the community's culture and its expressed needs.

To accurately identify these needs, understand the culture of the target community, and design an effective program, a team must be identified. Included must be members of the community to be served. These persons have insights into community values and norms and the evaluation methods that will be most acceptable to the target population. Here, science is a collaborative venture between the program developers, evaluators, and the communities they aid. This partnership elicits the input from the community regarding its needs, the goals and objectives of the program, the most effective intervention modalities to be employed, evaluation instrumentation and process, and mechanisms for the timely dissemination of evaluation findings.

Development refers to an ongoing process; it does not mean that changes cannot be made to a program once implementation has begun. Evaluation provides the mechanism for systematic feedback, through process and impact evaluation, that enables meaningful program modifications. AIDS service organizations must strive toward a planned evaluation strategy built into the design and development process prior to program implementation.

PROGRAM IMPLEMENTATION: A QUESTION OF REPLICABILITY

Evaluation of the effectiveness of an intervention must consider the replicability of results. Methodological issues often plague community-based AIDS researchers in their efforts to implement a successful program. These include lack of general populations; the lack of short, simple instruments that go beyond assessments of knowledge; lack of use of designs with control groups; reliance on participants' subjective self-reports; the tendency for respondents to give socially desirable responses; and low interview response, intervention participation, and retention rates. Practical problems faced by community-based organizations (CBOs) are: (1) fear that evaluation may be used punitively; (2) that their populations will be mere subjects for others' studies; (3) that rigid study protocols will hinder programmatic change; (4) inaccessibility to consultants; (5) inability to implement a rigorous evaluation on a shoestring budget; and (6) concerns about outreach staff's acceptability to respondents and their safety in community venues.

After launching innovative programs and determining whether they work, CBOs frequently do not give adequate thought to the long-term financing of programs. Consequently, timely exploration of other funding options is critical. Such options include developing community support for programs from community leaders, churches, and businesses; pooling resources and forming coalitions with other CBOs or institutions; and encouraging legislators to provide governmental support. One way to capture the attention of community and governmental officials is to disseminate program evaluation findings through written reports, media coverage, community forums, and presentation at HIV/AIDS-related conferences. The life of the program after evaluation must remain a primary goal.

EVALUATION

To date, many programs still lack well-defined development and evaluation components. Community-based organizations, however, are being increasingly required by funding agencies to evaluate their HIV/AIDS prevention programs. Support is often contingent on a sound, rigorous evaluation plan. For CBOs in their embryonic stages of development, this can be a double-edged sword. As CBOs struggle to provide concrete services to people with HIV infection or with high-risk behaviors in an era of shrinking dollars, diverting funds to the development and evaluation phases where tangible results may not be readily apparent may cause organizational tension. This sentiment may be further reinforced by a perceived dichotomy between humanistic-oriented research and

Gamble, V. N. (1993). A legacy of distrust: African Americans and medical research. *American Journal of Preventive Medicine, 9*, 35–38.

Gay Men's Health Crisis, Department of Education. (1989).

Gibbons, F. X., McGovern, P. G., & Lando, H. A. (1991). Relapse and risk perception among members of a smoking cessation clinic. *Health Psychology, 10*, 42–45.

Gielen, A. C., & Radius, S. (1984). Project KISS (kids in safety belts): Educational approaches and evaluation measures. *Health Education, 15*, 43–47.

Gillies, P. A., & Stork, A. (1988, June). Streetwize UK—A controlled trial of an AIDS education comic. Paper presented at the Fourth International Conference on AIDS, Stockholm, Sweden.

Gilmore, G. D. (1977). Needs assessment processes for community health education. *International Journal of Health Education, 20*(3), 164–173.

Ginzburg, H., French, J., Jackson, J., Hartsock, P. I., MacDonald, M., & Weiss, S. (1986). Health education and knowledge assessment of HTLV-III diseases among intravenous drug users. *Health Education Quarterly, 13*, 373–382.

Glanz, K., Lewis, F. M., & Rimer, B. K. (1990). *Health behavior and health education: Theory, research and practice.* San Francisco: Jossey-Bass.

Glanz, K., & Rimer, B. K. (1995). Theory at a glance: A guide for health promotion practice. Bethesda, MD: National Institutes of Health, National Cancer Institute.

Glaser, B. G., & Strauss, A. L. (1967). *The discovery of grounded theory: Strategies for qualitative research.* Chicago, IL: Aldine.

Goetz, J. P., & LeCompte, M. D. (1984). *Ethnography and qualitative design in educational research.* New York: Academic Press.

Goilav, C. (1988, June). Incidence of HIV infection and sexual practice in gay men in a low endemic area. Paper presented at the Fourth International Conference on AIDS, Stockholm, Sweden.

Goldfarb, E., Ehrhardt, A. A., Hoffman, S., Zawadski, R., & Elkin, S. (1993, October 15). HIV education: Evaluation of a behaviorally oriented intervention video, AIDS Is about Secrets. HIV Center for Clinical and Behavioral Studies at the New York State Psychiatric Institute. Draft of unpublished manuscript.

Goldfried, M. R., & D'Zurilla, T. J. (1969). A behavior-analytic model for assessing compliance. In C. D. Spielberger (Ed.), *Current topics in clinical psychology* (vol. 1, pp. 151–196). New York: Academic Press.

Goldman, J. A., & Harlow, L. L. (1993). Self-perception variables that mediate AIDS-preventive behavior in college students. *Health Psychology, 12*(6), 489–498.

Gordon, J. R. (1987, July). *Safer sex: A self-help manual.* Unpublished manuscript, University of Washington, School of Social Work, Seattle.

Gorman, D. M. (1993). A review of studies comparing checklist and interview methods of data collection in life event research. *Behavioral Medicine, 19*, 66–73.

Green, L. S., & Lewis, F. M. (1986). *Measurement and evaluation in health education and health promotion.* Palo Alto, CA: Mayfield.

Green, L. W., & Kreuter, M. W. (1991). *Health promotion planning: An educational and environmental approach.* Mountain View, CA: Mayfield.

Green, L. W., Wang, V. L., Deeds, S. G., Fisher, A., Windsor, R., Bennett, A., & Rogers, C. (1978). Guidelines for health education in maternal and child health programs. *International Journal of Health Education, 21*(suppl.), 1–33.

Grodin, M. A., Kaminow, P. V., & Sassower, R. (1986). Ethical issues in AIDS research. *QRB: Quality Review Bulletin, 12*, 347–352.

Guydish, J., Bucardo, J., Young, M., Woods, W., Grinstead, O., & Clark, W. (1993). Evaluating needle exchange: Are there negative effects? *AIDS, 7*, 871–876.

Guydish, J., Clark, G., Garcia, D., Downing, M., Case, P., & Sorensen, J. L. (1991). Evaluating needle exchange: Do distributed needles come back? *American Journal of Public Health, 81*, 617–619.

Hallal, J. C. (1982). The relationship of health beliefs, health locus of control, and self concept to the practice of breast self-examination in adult women. *Nursing Research, 31*, 137–142.

Hatch, J., Moss, N., Saran, A., Presley-Cantrell, L., & Malloy, C. (1993). Community research: Partnership in black communities. *American Journal of Preventive Medicine, 9*, 27–34.

Hays, R. B., & Peterson, J. L. (1994). HIV prevention for gay and bisexual men in metropolitan cities. In R. J.

DiClemente & J. L. Peterson (Eds.), *Preventing AIDS: Theories and methods in behavioral intervention* (pp. 267–296). New York: Plenum Press.

Hillman, E., Hovell, M. F., Williams, L., Hofstetter, R., & Burdyshaw, C. (1991). Pregnancy, STDs, and AIDS prevention: Evaluation of New Image teen theater. *AIDS Education and Prevention, 3,* 328–340.

Hingson, R. W., Strunin, L., Berlin, B. M., & Heeren, T. (1990). Beliefs about AIDS, use of alcohol and drugs and unprotected sex among Massachusetts adolescents. *American Journal of Public Health, 80,* 295–299.

HIV Center for Clinical and Behavioral Studies at the New York State Psychiatric Institute. (1989). *AIDS is about secrets,* video production. (Copyright, Research Foundation for Mental Hygiene, Inc.)

HIV Center for Clinical and Behavioral Studies at the New York State Psychiatric Institute. (1994). *Rompiendo el silencio/breaking the silence,* video production. (Copyright, Research Foundation for Mental Hygiene, Inc.)

Hochbaum, G. (1958). *Public participation in medical screening programs: A sociopsychological study.* Public Health Service publication No. 572. Rockville, MD: Public Health Service.

Hochbaum, G., Sorenson, J. R., & Lorig, K. (1992). Theory in health education practice. *Health Education Quarterly, 19,* 295–313.

Holland, J., Ramazanoglu, C., Scott, S., Sharpe, T., & Thomson, S. (1992). Risk, power and the possibility of pleasure: Young women and safer sex. *AIDS Care, 4,* 273–283.

Holt, R. R. (1982). Occupational stress. In R. Goldberger & S. Bresnitz (Eds.), *Handbook of stress: Theoretical and clinical aspects* (pp. 419–439). New York: Free Press.

Holtgrave, D. R. (1994). Cost analysis and HIV prevention interventions. *American Psychologist, 49,* 1088–1089.

Huang, K. H. C., Watters, J. K., & Case, P. (1989, June). Compliance with AIDS prevention measures among intravenous drug users: Health beliefs or social/environmental factors? Paper M.D.O.5 presented at the Fifth International Conference on AIDS, Montreal, Canada.

Huberman, A. M., & Miles, M. B. (1994). Data management and analysis methods. In N. K. Denzin & Y. S. Lincoln (Eds.), *Handbook of qualitative research* (pp. 428–444). Thousand Oaks, CA: Sage.

Isbell, M. (1993). AIDS and public health: The enduring relevance of a communitarian approach to disease prevention. *AIDS and Public Policy Journal, 8,* 157–177.

Jackson, J., & Rotkiewicz, L. (1987, June). A coupon program: AIDS education and drug treatment. Paper presented at the Third International Conference on AIDS, Washington, DC.

Janz, N. K., & Becker, M. H. (1984). The health belief model: A decade later. *Health Education Quarterly, 11,* 1–47.

Janz, N. K., Zimmerman, M. A., Wren, P. A., Israel, B. A., Freudenberg, N., & Carter, R. J. (1996). Evaluation of 37 AIDS prevention projects: Successful approaches and barriers to program effectiveness. *Health Education Quarterly, 23,* 80–97.

Jemmott, L. S., & Jemmott, J. (1991). Applying the theory of reasoned action to AIDS risk behavior: Condom use among black women. *Nursing Research, 40*(4), 228–234.

John Snow, Inc. (1993). The formation and operation of coalitions to provide health care services to people with HIV illness: Analytic synopsis. Washington, DC: U.S. Department of Health and Human Services.

Jones, J. H. (1993). *Bad blood: The Tuskegee syphilis experiment* (2nd ed.). New York: Free Press.

Joseph, J. D., Montgomery, S. B., Emmons, C. A., Kirscht, J. P., Kessler, R. C., Ostrow, D. G., Wortman, C. B., O'Brien, K., Eller, M., & Eschleman, S. (1987). Magnitude and determinants of behavioral risk reduction: Longitudinal analysis of a cohort at risk for AIDS. *Psychology and Health, 1,* 73–96.

Kahn, R., & Cannell, C. (1957). *The dynamics of interviewing.* New York: John Wiley.

Kalton, G. (1983). *Introduction to survey sampling.* Beverly Hills, CA: Sage.

Kaluzny, A. D, & Hernandez, S. R. (1988). Organization change and function. In S. M. Shortell and A. D. Kaluzny (Eds.), *Health care management: A text in organization theory and behavior* (2nd ed., pp. 379–417). New York: Wiley.

Kaplan, E. H. (1991). Evaluating needle-exchange programs via syringe tracking and testing (STT). *AIDS and Public Policy Journal, 6,* 109–115.

Kaplan, E. H., & Heimer, R. (1995). HIV incidence among New Haven needle exchange participants: Updated estimates from syringe tracking and testing data. *Journal of Acquired Immune Deficiency Syndromes and Human Retrovirology, 10,* 175–176.

Manalansan, M. F., IV. (1992b, May). Telephone survey of service providers in four boroughs: Second phase. Unpublished manuscript, Gay Men's Health Crisis, New York.

Manalansan, M. F., IV. (1992c). Subway ad campaign audience survey: Third phase. Unpublished manuscript, Gay Men's Health Crisis, New York.

Manalansan, M. F., IV, Frederick, R. J., Humes, S., Moraes, A. M., & McDaniel, B. (1993). An evaluation of an HIV secondary prevention media campaign focusing on PCP prophylaxis. Unpublished manuscript, Gay Men's Health Crisis, New York.

Mantell, J. E. (1990). Interview guide for focus groups on HIV knowledge, testing and partner notification. New York: The New York City Department of Health.

Mantell, J. E., & DiVittis, A. T. (1989). Rand Corporation modified social support scale, CDC Cooperative Agreement #U62/CCU201065. Gay Men's Health Crisis final report to the Centers for Disease Control. New York: Gay Men's Health Crisis, HIV Behavioral Research Program.

Mantell, J. E., & DiVittis, A. T. (1990, Summer). Evaluating AIDS prevention: Contributions of multiple disciplines. *New Directions for Program Evaluation, 46,* 87–98.

Mantell, J. E., DiVittis, A. T., Kochems, L., & Ostfield, M. (1989a). Final report: HIV risk reduction interventions targeted to groups with high-risk behavior (CDC Cooperative Agreement #U62/CCU201065). New York: Gay Men's Health Crisis.

Mantell, J. E., DiVittis, A. T., Kochems, L., & Ostfield, M. (1989b). Project HEART (CDC Cooperative Agreement #U62/CCU201065). New York: Gay Men's Health Crisis.

Mantell, J. E., Karim, Q. A., & Scheepers, E. (1996, July). Developing a training program in female controlled methods of HIV prevention for South African health care providers. Paper presented at the XI International Conference on AIDS, Toronto, Canada.

Mantell, J. E., Kenny, M. E., & Cortez, N. (1989c). *Ethnographic interview guide for men.* New York: New York City Department of Health, Perinatal HIV Prevention Demonstration Project.

Mantell, J. E., Ramos, S. E., DiVittis, A. T., & Whittier, D. (1989d). Perinatal HIV Prevention Project, Qualitative Interview Guide. Prevention of perinatal HIV infection demonstration project, Medical and Health Research Association of New York City.

Mantell, J. E., Ramos, S. E., Karp, G. B., & Roman, R. J. (1995, July). Prevention of perinatal HIV infection demonstration project, Medical and Health Research Association of New York City, Final Report to the Centers for Disease Control and Prevention, Cooperative Agreement Number U6621CCU303330.

Mantell, J. E., Rapkin, B., Tross, S. E., & Ortíz-Torres, B. (1992). Cultural Network Project, Baseline Instrument, Medical and Health Research Association of New York City.

Mantell, J. E., Schinke, S. P., & Akabas, S. H. (1988). Women and AIDS prevention. *Journal of Primary Prevention, 9,* 18–40.

Marks, A. S., & Downes, G. M. (1991). Informal sector shops and AIDS prevention. *South African Medical Journal, 79,* 496–499.

Markus, G. A. (1990). Toward a "critical mass" theory of interactive media. In J. Falk & C. Steinfield (Eds.), *Organizations and communication technology* (pp. 194–1228). Newbury Park, CA: Sage.

Marlatt, G. A. (1973, April). A comparison of aversive conditioning procedures in the treatment of alcoholism. Paper presented at the Annual Meeting of the Western Psychological Association, Anaheim, CA.

Marlatt, G. A., Curry, S., & Gordon, J. R. (1988). A longitudinal analysis of unaided smoking cessation. *Journal of Consulting and Clinical Psychology, 56*(5), 715–720.

Marlatt, G. A., & Gordon, J. R. (Eds.). (1985). *Relapse prevention: Maintenance strategies in the treatment of addictive behaviors.* New York: Guilford Press.

Marsella, A. J., & Dash-Scheuer, A. (1988). Coping, culture, and healthy human development. In P. R. Dasen, J. W. Berry, & N. Sartorius. (Eds.), *Health and cross-cultural psychology* (pp. 162–178). Newbury Park, CA: Sage.

Marshall, C., & Rossman, G. B. (1989). *Designing qualitative research.* Newbury Park, CA: Sage.

Marshall, C., & Rossman, G. B. (1995). *Designing qualitative research* (2nd ed.). Thousand Oaks, CA: Sage.

Martin, J. L. (1985). The impact of AIDS on gay male sexual behavior patterns in New York City. *American Journal of Public Health, 77,* 578–581.

Mays, V. M., & Cochran, S. D. (1988). Issues in the perceptions of AIDS risk and risk reduction activities of black and Hispanic/Latina women. *American Psychologist, 43,* 949–957.

McAlister, A., Puska, P., Salomen, J. T., & Koskela, K. (1982). Theory and action for health promotion: Illustrations from the North Karelia Project. *American Journal of Public Health, 72,* 43–50.

McCoy, H. V., & Inciardi, J. A. (1993). Women and AIDS: Social determinants of sex-related activities. *Women and Health, 20,* 69–86.

McCrae, F. A., Hill, D. J., St. John, D. J., Ambikapathy, A., & Garner, J. F. (1984). Predicting colon cancer screening behavior from health beliefs. *Preventive Medicine, 13,* 115–126.

McElroy, K. R., Kegler, M., Steckler, A., Burdine, J. M., & Wisotzky, M. (1994). Community coalitions for health promotion: Summary and further reflections. *Health Education Research: Theory and Practice, 9,* 1–11.

McGinn, T., Bamba, A., & Balma, M. (1989). Male knowledge, use and attitudes regarding family planning in Burkino Faso. *International Family Planning Perspectives, 15,* 84–87.

McKeganey, N., Barnard, M., Bloor, M., & Leyland, A. (1990). Injecting drug use and female street-working prostitution in Glasgow. *AIDS, 4,* 1153–1155.

McKillip, J. (1987). *Needs analysis. Tool for the human services and education.* Newbury Park, CA: Sage.

McKinley, J. C. (1996, April 7). A ray of light in African struggle with AIDS. *The New York Times,* pp. 1, 6.

McKusick, L., Coates, T. J., Morin, S. F., Pollack, L. & Hoff, C. (1990). Longitudinal predictors of reduction in unprotected anal intercourse among gay men in San Francisco: The AIDS Behavior Research Project. *American Journal of Public Health, 80,* 978–983.

McKusick, L., Horstman, W., & Coates, T. J. (1985). AIDS and sexual behavior of gay men in San Francisco. *American Journal of Public Health, 75,* 493–496.

McLaws, M. L, Oldenburg, B., Ross, M. W., & Cooper, D. A. (1990). Sexual behavior in AIDS-related research: Reliability and validity of recall and diary measures. *The Journal of Sex Research, 27,* 265–281.

Melton, G. B., & Gray, J. N. (1988). Ethical dilemmas in AIDS research: Individual privacy and public health. *American Psychologist, 43,* 60–64.

Menaghan, E. (1984). Measuring coping effectiveness: A panel analysis of marital problems and coping efforts. *Journal of Health and Social Behavior, 23,* 220–234.

Menzel, H., & Katz, E. (1955). Social relations and innovations in the medical profession: The epidemiology of a new drug. *Public Opinion Quarterly, 19,* 337–352.

Miles, M. B., & Huberman, A. M. (1994). *Qualitative data analysis* (2nd ed., pp. 1–15). Thousand Oaks, CA: Sage.

Miller, J. G. (1989). A roving clinic: Community outreach to gay and bisexual men. *Public Health Reports, 104,* 88.

Miller, R. L., & Cassel, B. J. (in press). Ongoing evaluation in AIDS service organizations: Building meaningful evaluation activities. *Journal of Prevention in the Community.*

Miller, R. L., Holmes, J. M., & Auerbach, M. I. (1992, November). Psychological environments of AIDS volunteers: Perceptions of workplace climate. Paper presented at the Annual Meeting of the American Public Health Association, Washington, DC.

Miller, S. (1995). *A planning guide for intervention decisions.* New York: HIV Center for Clinical and Behavioral Studies at the New York State Psychiatric Institute.

Miller, T. E., Booraem, C., Flowers, J. V., & Iversen, A. E. (1990). Changes in knowledge, attitudes, and behavior as a result of a community-based AIDS prevention program. *AIDS Education and Prevention, 2,* 12–23.

Moher, D., Dulberg, C. S., & Wells, G. A. (1994). Statistical power, sample size, and their reporting in randomized controlled trials. *Journal of the American Medical Association, 272,* 122–124.

Montgomery, S., Joseph, J., Becker, M., Ostrow, D., Kessler, R., & Kirscht, J. (1989). The health belief model in understanding compliance with preventive recommendations for AIDS: How useful? *AIDS Education and Prevention, 1*(4), 303–33.

Moreau, D. (1993). *AIDS prevention for girls in therapy for depression study.* New York: HIV Center for Clinical and Behavioral Studies at the New York State Psychiatric Institute.

Morgan, D. L. (1988). *Focus groups as qualitative research.* Newbury Park, CA: Sage.

Morgan, D. L. (1993). Future directions for focus groups. In D.L. Morgan (Ed.), *Successful focus groups. Advancing the state of the art.* (pp. 228–244). Newbury Park, CA: Sage.

Mulleady, G., Green, J., Roderick, P., Flanagan, D., Burnyeat, S., Wade, B., Clarke, H., & McAught, A. (1988, June). Evaluation of a syringe exchange scheme. Paper presented at the Fourth International Conference on AIDS, Stockholm, Sweden.

Mushkin, P. R., & Stevens, L. A. (1990). An AIDS educational program for third-year medical students. *General Hospital Psychiatry, 12,* 390–395.

National Institute on Drug Abuse, Community Research Branch. (1988, December). AIDS initial assessment questionnaire, AIA 8.0. National AIDS Demonstration Research Project.

Newman, L. F. (1987, September). Ethnographic approaches to AIDS: Understanding contact, transmission and prevention. Paper presented at the NIMH/NIDA Workshop on Women and AIDS: Promoting Healthy Behaviors, Bethesda, MD.

New York State Department of Health AIDS Institute (1994, June). Request for concept papers. Intervention and evaluation of HIV risk reduction strategies targeted to women.

New York Times (1996, June 28). Doctors back AIDS tests for pregnant women. *The New York Times*, page A20.

Nyamathi, A. M., Leake, B., Flaskerud, J., Lewis, C., & Bennett, C. (1993). Outcomes of specialized and traditional AIDS counseling programs for impoverished women of color. *Research in Nursing and Health, 16*, 11–21.

O'Leary, A. (1985). Self-efficacy and health. *Behavior Research Therapy, 23*, 427–451.

O'Leary, A., Goodhart, F., & Jemmott, L. S. (1991). Social cognitive theory and AIDS prevention on the college campus: Implications for intervention. Unpublished manuscript. New Brunswick, NJ: Rutgers University.

O'Reilly, K. R., & Higgins, D. L. (1991). AIDS community demonstration projects for HIV prevention among hard-to-reach groups. *Public Health Reports, 106*, 714–720.

Ortíz-Torres, B., & Ehrhardt, A. A. (1995). Evaluation and dissemination of an AIDS educational video for Latinas: Breaking the silence. Unpublished paper, HIV Center for Clinical and Behavioral Studies at the New York State Psychiatric Institute, New York.

Ortíz-Torres, B., Ehrhardt, A. A., Van Dommelen, E., Del Carmen Rivera, M., & Rivera, M. (1996, July). Women's social networks as a vehicle for empowerment: A diffusion-of-innovation approach to encourage risk reduction behaviors among Latinas. Poster No. Tu.D.2750 presented at the Eleventh International Conference on AIDS, Vancouver, British Columbia.

Ortíz-Torres, B., Rapkin, B., Mantell, J. E., & Tross, S. (1992, July). Is transculturation related to sexual risk behavior among Latinas? Poster presented at the Eighth International Conference on AIDS, Amsterdam, The Netherlands.

Padilla, A. M., & Salgado de Snyder, V. N. (1992). Hispanics: What the culturally informed evaluator needs to know. In M. A. Orlandi, E. R. Weston, & L. G. Epstein (Eds.), *Cultural competence for evaluators: A guide for alcohol and other drug abuse prevention practitioners working with ethnic/racial communities.* (pp. 117–146). Rockville, MD: US Department of Health and Human Services.

Parker, W. (1995). Society for Family Health adolescent programme and AMREP in conjunction with youth of the Youth Leadership Development Programme. Ipelegeng-Soweto, Republic of South Africa: Media Product Research.

Parl, B. (1967). *Basic statistics.* Garden City, NY: Doubleday.

Patton, M. (1978). Utilization-focused evaluation. Beverly Hills, CA: Sage.

Pear, R. (1992, December 29). States face drop in federal backing of AIDS prevention. *The New York Times*, pp. A1, A10.

Perloff, R. M., & Pettey, G. (1991). Designing an AIDS information campaign to reach intravenous drug users and sex partners. *Public Health Reports, 109*(4), 460–463.

Peterson, D. R. (1979). Assessing interpersonal relationships in natural settings. *Methods for studying person situation interactions. New directions for methodology of behavioral science 2*, 33–54.

Peterson, J. L., & Marin, G. (1988). Issues in the prevention of AIDS among black and hispanic men. *American Psychologist, 43*, 871–877.

Petosa, R., & Jackson, K. (1991). Using the health belief model to predict safer sex intentions among adolescents. *Health Education Quarterly, 18*, 463–476.

Phillips, E. L. (1985). Social skills. History and prospect. In L. L'Abate & M. A. Milan (Eds.), *Handbook of social skills training and research* (pp. 3–21). New York: Wiley-Interscience.

Pithers, W. D., Marques, J. K., Gibat, C. C., & Marlatt, G. A. (1983). Relapse prevention with sexual aggressives: A self-control model of treatment and maintenance of change. In J. G. Greer & I. Stuart (Eds.), *The sexual aggressor: Current perspectives on treatment* (pp. 214–239) New York: Van Nostrand Reinhold.

Porter, L. W., & Steers, R. M. (1973). Organizational, work and personal factors in employee turnover and absenteeism. *Psychological Bulletin, 80*, 151–176.

Probart, C. K. (1989). A preliminary investigation using drama in community AIDS education. *AIDS Education and Prevention, 1*, 268–276.

Prochaska, J. O., & DiClemente, C. C. (1983). Stages and processes of self-change of smoking: Toward an integrative model of change. *Journal of Consulting and Clinical Psychology, 51*, 390–395.

Prochaska, J. O., & DiClemente, C. C. (1986). Toward a comprehensive model of change. In W. R. Miller & N. Healther (Eds.), *Treating addictive behaviors* (pp. 3–27) New York: Plenum Press.

Prochaska, J. O., & DiClemente, C. C. (1992). Stages of change in the modification of problem behaviors. In M. Hersen, R. M. Eisler, & P. M. Miller (Eds.), *Progress in behavior modification* (pp. 184–218). Sycamore, IL: Sycamore Press.

Prochaska, J. O., Redding, C. A., Harlow, L. L., Rossi, J. S., & Velicer, W. F. (1994). The transtheoretical model of change and HIV prevention: A review. *Health Education Quarterly, 21*, 471–486.

Psychosocial/Qualitative Assessment Core & Carballo-Dieguez, A. (1994, August). *Puerto Rican men's study*. New York: HIV Center for Clinical and Behavioral Studies at the New York Psychiatric Institute.

Rand Corporation. (1988). The role of social support and life stress events in the use of mental health services. Behavioral Sciences Department, Santa Monica, California. *Social Science and Medicine, 27*(12), 1393–1400.

Randall-David, E. (1994). *Culturally competent HIV counseling*. Washington, DC: National Hemophilia Program, Maternal and Child Health Bureau, Health Resources and Services Administration.

Rapkin, B. D. (1995, October). Analyzing your data at the group and individual levels. The female condom as a women-controlled protective method workshop, for AIDSCAP/FHI. HIV Center for Clinical and Behavioral Studies at the New York State Psychiatric Institute, New York.

Rapkin, B. D., & Smith, M. Y. (1992). *Activities for Life Project*. New York: Memorial Sloan-Kettering Cancer Center, Department of Psychiatry.

Rapkin, B. D., Smith, M. Y., DuMont, K., Correa, A., Palmer, S., & Cohen, S. (1994). Development of the idiographic functional status assessment: A measure of the personal goals and goal attainment activities of people with AIDS. *Psychology and Health 9*, 111–129.

Reinsich, J. M., Sanders, S. A., & Ziemba-Davis, M. (1988). The study of sexual behavior in relation to the transmission of the human immunodeficiency virus. *American Psychologist, 43*, 921–927.

Research Triangle Institute. (1995, January/February/March). Delicate subjects. *Research Triangle Institute Hypotenuse*, pp. 2–5.

Rhodes, T., & Holland, J. (1992). Outreach as a strategy for HIV prevention: Aims and practice. *Health Education Research, 7*, 533–546.

Richards, T. J., & Richards, L. (1994). Using computers in qualitative research. In N. K. Denzin & Y. S. Lincoln (Eds.), *Handbook of qualitative research* (pp. 445–462). Thousand Oaks, CA: Sage.

Rickert, V. I., Gottlieb, A., & Jay, M. S. (1990). A comparison of three clinic-based AIDS education programs on female adolescents' knowledge, attitudes and behavior. *Journal of Adolescent Health Care, 11*, 298–303.

Ripptoe, P. A., & Rogers, R. W. (1987). Effects of components of protection-motivation theory on adaptive and maladaptive coping with a health threat. *Journal of Personality and Social Psychology, 52*, 596–604.

Robert, B., and Rosser, S. (1990). Evaluation of the efficacy of AIDS education interventions for homosexually active men. *Health Education Research, 5*, 299–308.

Rogers, E. M. (1983). *Diffusion of innovations* (3rd ed.). New York: Free Press.

Rogers, R. W. (1975). A protection motivation theory of fear appeals and attitude change. *Journal of Psychology, 91*, 93–114.

Rogers, R. W., & Mewborn, C. R. (1976). Fear appeals and attitude change: Effects of a threat's seriousness, probability of occurrence, and the efficacy of coping responses. *Journal of Personality and Social Psychology, 34*, 54–61.

Rogers, R. W., & Shoemaker, F. (1971). *Communication of innovations*. New York: Free Press.

Rosenstock, I. M. (1966). Why people use health services. *Milbank Memorial Fund Quarterly, 44*, 94–124.

Rosenstock, I. M. (1974). The health belief model and personal health behavior. *Health Education Monographs, 2*, 220–243.

Rosenstock, I. M., Strecher, V. J., & Becker, M. H. (1988). Social learning and the health belief model. *Health Education Quarterly, 15*(2), 175–183.

Rosenstock, I. M., Strecher, V. J., & Becker, M. H. (1994). The health belief model and HIV behavior change. In R. J. DiClemente & J. L. Peterson (Eds.), *Preventing AIDS: Theories and methods of behavioral interventions* (pp. 5–24). New York: Plenum Press.

Ross, M. W., & McLaws, M. L. (1992). Subjective norms about condoms are better predictors of use and intention to use than attitudes. *Health Education Research, 7,* 335–339.

Rossi, P. H. (1993). *Evaluation: A systematic approach.* Newbury Park, CA: Sage.

Rothenberg, R. B. (1993). Confounding in community interventions. *American Journal of Preventive Medicine, 9,* 372–377.

Rotter, J. (1966). Generalized expectancies for internal versus external control of reinforcement. *Psychological Monographs, 80.*

Rudd, R. E., Allender, J., Mueller, C., Cole, R., Auerbach, M. I., Henry, R., Seechuck, R., Rhodes, F., Connell, D., Ager, J., Null, C., & Stephenson, J. (1994). Health-related training programs for health care professionals: Findings from a collaborative assessment. *AIDS Education and Prevention, 6,* 283–295.

Rudd, R. E., Henry, R., Cole, R., Rhodes, F., Seechuk, K., Auerbach, M. I., Connell, D., Allender, J., Mueller, W., Ager, J., Null, C., & Stephenson, J. (1993). *Evaluator collaboration across diverse AIDS-related education programs. Evaluation Practice, 14*(3), 243–251.

Rugg, D. L. (1990, Summer). AIDS prevention: A public health psychology perspective. *New Directions for Program Evaluation, 46,* 7–22.

Rugg, D. L., MacGowan, R. J., Stark, K. A., & Swanson, N. M. (1991). Evaluating the CDC program for HIV counseling and testing. *Public Health Reports, 106,* 708–713.

Runge, C., Prentice-Dunn, S., & Scogin, F. (1993). Protection motivation theory and alcohol use attitudes among older adults. *Psychology Reports, 73*(1), 96–98.

Runkle, C. (1990, June). The use of focus groups for coalition and organizational support for health education. Paper presented at the Mid-year Scientific Conference of the Society for Public Health Education, Portland, Maine.

Schaalma, H. P., Kok, G. J., Braeken, D., Schoopman, M., & Deven, F. (1991). Sex and AIDS education for adolescents. *Tijdschfirt voor Seksuologie (Journal for Sexology), 15,* 140–149.

Schaalma, H., Kok, G., & Peters, L. (1993). Determinants of consistent condom use by adolescents: The impact of experience of sexual intercourse. *Health Education Research, 8*(2), 225–269.

Schensul, J. J., & Schensul, S. L. (1990, Summer). Ethnographic evaluation of AIDS prevention programs: Better data for better programs. *New Directions for Program Evaluation, 46,* 51–62.

Schinke, S. P., Gordon, A. N., & Weston, E. R. (1990). Self-instruction to prevent HIV infection among African-American and Hispanic-American adolescents. *Journal of Consulting and Clinical Psychology, 58,* 432–436.

Schlundt, D. G., & McFall, R. M. (1985). New directions in the assessment of social competence and social skills. In L. L'Abate & M. A. Milan (Eds.), *Handbook of social skills training and research* (pp. 22–49). New York: Wiley-Interscience.

Schoonover, S. C., Bassuk, E. L., Smith, R., & Gaskill, D. (1983). The use of videotape programs to teach interpersonal skills. *Journal of Medical Education, 58,* 804–810.

Schuh, A. (1967). The predictability of employee tenure: A review of the literature. *Personnel Psychology, 20,* 133–152.

Scrimshaw, S. C., Carballo, M., Ramos, L., & Blair, B. A. (1991). The AIDS rapid anthropological assessment procedures: A tool for health education planning and evaluation. *Health Education Quarterly, 18,* 111–123.

Sechrest, L., Ametrano, I. M., & Ametrano, D. A. (1982). Program evaluation. In J. R. McNamara & A. G. Barclay (Eds.), *Critical issues, developments, and trends in professional psychology* (pp. 190–226). New York: Praeger.

Sechrest, L., Ametrano, I. M., & Ametrano, D. A. (1983). Evaluations of social programs. In C.E. Walker (Ed.), *The handbook of clinical psychology* (vol. 1, pp. 129–166). Homewood, IL: Dow Jones-Irwin.

Sechrest, L. C., & Yeaton, W. E. (1981). Assessing the effectiveness of social programs: Methodological and conceptual issues. *New Directions for Program Evaluation, 9,* 41–55.

Seeley, J. A., Kengeya-Kayonda, J. F., & Mulder, D. W. (1992). Community-based HIV/AIDS research— Whither community participation? Unresolved problems in a research programme in rural Uganda. *Social Science and Medicine, 34,* 1089–1095.

Sejwac, R., Ajzen, I. & Fishbein, M. (1980). Predicting and understanding weight loss: Intentions, behaviors and outcomes. In I. Ajzen & M. Fishbein (Eds.), *Understanding attitudes and predicting social behavior* (pp. 101–112). Englewood Cliffs, NJ: Prentice-Hall.

Sherr, L., & McCreaner, A. (1989). Summary evaluation of the national AIDS counselling training unit in the U.K. *Counselling Psychology Quarterly, 2,* 21–32.

Shulman, L. C., Mantell, J. E., Eaton, C., & Sorrell, S. (1990). HIV-related disorders, needle users, and the social services. In C.G. Leukefeld, R.J. Battjes, & Z. Amsel (Eds.), *AIDS and intravenous drug use: Future directions for community-based prevention research.* (pp. 254–275). Washington, DC: National Institute on Drug Abuse Research Monograph 93. DHHS Pub. No. (ADM) 90-1627.

Siegel, K., Grodsky, P. B., & Herman, A. (1986). AIDS risk reduction guidelines: A review and analysis. *Journal of Community Health, 11,* 233–243.

Sikkema, K. J., Winett, R. A., & Lombard, D. N. A. (1995a). Development and evaluation of an HIV-risk reduction program for female college students. *AIDS Education and Prevention, 7,* 145–159.

Sikkema, K. J., Kelly, J. A., Heckman, T. G., Wagstaff, D. A., Crumble, D. A., Cargill, V. A., Mercer, M. B., Solomon, L., Perry, M. J., Roffman, R. A., Norman, A. D., Winett, R. A., & Anderson, E. (1995b, February). Urban Women's Health Project, Community intervention to reduce HIV risk behavior for women in housing developments, Center for AIDS Intervention Research, Medical College of Wisconsin, NIMH Center Grant #P30-MH52776 and Grant #R01-MH42908-07. Presentation at HIV rounds, HIV Center for Clinical and Behavioral Studies at the New York State Psychiatric Institute.

Siska, M., Jason, J., Murdoch, P., Shan Yang, W., & Donovan, R. J. (1992). Recall of AIDS public service announcements and their impact on the ranking of AIDS as a national problem. *American Journal of Public Health, 82,* 1029–1032.

Skinner, D., Metcalf, C. A., Seager, J. R., de Swardt, J. S., & Laubscher, J. A. (1991). An evaluation of an education programme on HIV infection using puppetry and street theatre. *AIDS Care, 3,* 317–329.

Slater, M. D., & Flora, J. A. (1991). Health lifestyles: Audience segmentation analysis for public health interventions. *Health Education Quarterly, 18,* 221–233.

Solomon, M. Z., & DeJong, W. (1986). Recent sexually transmitted disease prevention efforts and their implications for AIDS health education. *Health Education Quarterly, 13,* 301–316.

Solomon, M. Z., & DeJong, W. (1989). Preventing AIDS and other STDs through condom promotion: A patient education intervention. *American Journal of Public Health, 79,* 453–458.

Spivak, G., Platt, J. J., & Shure, M. B. (1976). *The problem solving approach to adjustment.* San Francisco: CA: Jossey-Bass.

Spradley, J. P. (1979). *The ethnographic interview.* New York: Holt, Rinehart and Winston.

Spradley, J. P., & McCurdy, D. W. (1972). *The cultural experience.* Chicago, IL: Science Research Associates.

Steckler, A., McLeroy, K. R., Goodman, R. M., Bird, G. T., & McCormick, L. (1992). Toward integrating qualitative and quantitative methods: An introduction. *Health Education Quarterly, 19,* 1–8.

Stewart, D. W. & Shamdasani, P. N. (1990). *Focus groups: Theory and practice.* Newbury Park, CA.: Sage.

Stimson, G. V. (1989). Syringe-exchange programmes for injecting drug users. *AIDS, 3,* 253–260.

Strecher, V. J., DeVellis, B. M., Becker, M., & Rosenstock, I. M. (1986). The role of self-efficacy in achieving health behavior. *Health Education Quarterly, 13,* 73–91.

Stryker, J., Coates, T. J., DeCarlo, P., Haynes-Sanstad, K., Shriver, M., & Makadon, H. J. (1995). Prevention of HIV infection. Looking back, looking ahead. *Journal of the American Medical Association, 273,* 1143–1148.

Sue, D., Arredondo, P., & McDavis, R. (1992). Multicultural counseling competencies and standards: A call to the profession. *Journal of Counseling and Development, 70,* 477–486.

Temmerman, M., Moses, S., Kiragu, D., Fusallah, S., Wamola, I. A., & Piot, P. (1990). Impact of a single session post-partum counselling of HIV-infected women on their subsequent reproductive behaviour. *AIDS Care, 2,* 247–251.

Thomas, S. (1991). Evaluation and risk reduction projects in ethnic and racial minority communities. *Journal of Health Education, 22,* 24–29.

Thomas, S., & Morgan, C. (1991). Evaluation of community based AIDS education and risk reduction projects in ethnic and racial minority communities: A survey project funded by the US Public Health Service. *Program Planning and Evaluation, 14,* 247–255.

Thomas, S. B., & Quinn, S. C. (1991). The Tuskegee syphilis study, 1932 to 1972: Implications for HIV education and AIDS risk reduction programs in the black community. *American Journal of Public Health, 81*, 1498–1505.

Tichy, N. M., & Beckhard, R. (1982). Organizational development for health care organizations. In N. Margulis & J. D. Adams (Eds.), *Organizational development in health care organizations*. Reading, MA: Addison-Wesley.

Unger, D. G., & Wandersman, L. P. (1985). Social support and adolescent mothers: Action research contributions to theory and application. *Journal of Social Issues, 41*, 29–45.

US Centers for Disease Control (1991a). *America responds to AIDS materials catalog*. Rockville, MD: National AIDS Clearinghouse.

US Centers for Disease Control and Prevention, Division of STD/HIV, AIDS Community Demonstration Projects, HIV Prevention Interventions (1991b, April 23). Brief street intercept.

US Conference of Mayors. (1989, August). *Teen teatro: East Los Angeles Rape Hotline, HIV Education Case Studies*, No. 1, pp. 1–12. A review of community based HIV education programs funded by the United States Conference of Mayors.

US Conference of Mayors. (1990, December). Evaluation for HIV/AIDS Prevention Programs. *Technical Assistance Reports*. AIDS/HIV Program. US Conference of Mayors, pp. 1–12.

US Conference of Mayors. (1994, June). Assessing the HIV prevention of gay and bisexual men of color. *AIDS Information Exchange, 11*, 1–11.

US General Accounting Office. (1988, September). AIDS education: Reaching populations at higher risk. Report to the Chairman, Committee on Governmental Affairs, US Senate GAO/PEMD-88-35.

US Office of Technology Assessment. Congress of the United States. (1995, September). The effectiveness of AIDS prevention efforts. OTA-BP-H-172.

Valdiserri, R. O., Lyter, D. W., Leviton, L. C., Callahan, C. M., Kingsley, L. A., & Rinaldo, C. R. (1989). AIDS prevention in homosexual and bisexual men: Results of a randomized trial evaluating two risk reduction interventions. *AIDS, 3*, 21–26.

Van de Ven, A. L. H., & Delbecq, A. L. (1972). The nominal group as a research instrument for exploratory studies. *American Journal of Public Health, 62*, 337–342.

Van den Hoek, J. A. R., Van Haastrecht, H. J. A., & Coutinho, R. A. (1989). Risk reduction among intravenous drug users in Amsterdam under the influence of AIDS. *American Journal of Public Health, 79*, 1355–1357.

Van der Velde, F. W., & Van der Pligt, J. (1991). AIDS-related health behavior: Coping, protection motivation and previous behavior. *Journal of Behavioral Medicine, 14* (5), 429–451.

Walkey, F. H., Taylor, A. J. W., & Green, D. E. (1990). Attitudes to AIDS: A comparative analysis of a new and negative stereotype. *Social Science and Medicine, 30*, 549–552.

Wallack, L. (1990). Two approaches to health promotion in the mass media. *World Health Forum, 11*, 143–153.

Walter, H. J., Vaughan, R. D., Gladis, M. M., Ragin, D. F., Kasen, S., & Cohall, A. T. (1992). Factors associated with AIDS risk behavior among high school students in AIDS epicenter. *American Journal of Public Health, 82*, 528–532.

Wendt, E. (Ed.) (1965). Evaluating educational research. In *A cross-section of educational research* (pp. 1–13). New York: McKay.

Wiebel, W. W. (1988). Combining ethnographic and epidemiologic methods in targeted AIDS interventions: The Chicago model. In R. J. Battjes & R. W. Pickens (Eds.), *Needle sharing among intravenous drug users: National and international perspectives* (pp. 137–150). NIDA Research Monograph No. 80. Washington, DC: US Government Printing Office.

Wilkerson, I. (1991, June 3). Medical experiment still haunts blacks. *The New York Times*, p. A12.

Williams, D. G., Best, J. A., Taylor, D. W., Gilbert, J. R., Wilsen, D. M. C., Lindsay, E. A., & Singer, J. (1990). A systematic approach for using qualitative methods in primary prevention research. *Medical Anthropology Quarterly, 4*, 391–409.

Winett, R. A., Altman, D. G., & King, A. C. (1990). Conceptual and strategic foundations for effective media campaigns for preventing the spread of HIV infection. *Evaluation and Program Planning, 13* (1), 91–104.

Winett, R. A., King, A. C., & Altman, D. G. (1989). Incentives in health promotion: A theoretical framework and applications. In R. A. Winett (Ed.), *Health psychology and public health: An integrative approach* (pp. 71–92) New York: Pergamon Press.

World Health Organization (1989). Acquired immunodeficiency syndrome (AIDS): Consensus statement from consultation on partner notification for preventing HIV transmission. *Weekly Epidemiological Record, 64,* 77–82.

World Health Organization Global Programme on AIDS (1993). Social marketing campaign swaps condoms for bottle tops. *Global AIDS News, 2,* 11.

Wyatt, G. E. (1987, September). Ethnic and culture differences in women's sexual behavior. Paper presented at the NIMH/NIDA Workshop on Women and AIDS: Promoting Healthy Behaviors, Bethesda, MD.

Wyld, D. C., & Hallock, D. E. (1989). Advertising's response to the AIDS crisis: The role of social marketing. *AIDS and Public Policy Journal, 4,* 193–205.

Yeaton, W. H., & Sechrest, L. (1987). No-difference research. In D. S. Corray, H. S. Bloom, & R. J. Light (Eds.), *Evaluation practice in review: New directions for program evaluation* (pp. 67–82). San Francisco: Jossey-Bass.

Zabin, L., & Clark, S. D., Jr. (1981). Why they delay: A study of teenage family planning clinic patients. *Family Planning Perspectives, 13,* 205–217.

Recommended Readings

Agar, M. H. (1986). *Speaking of ethnography.* Beverly Hills, CA: Sage.

AIDSTECH (1992). *Tools for project evaluation: A guide for evaluating AIDS prevention interventions.* Durham, NC: AIDSTECH.

Berk, R. A., & Rossi, P. H. (1990). *Thinking about program evaluation.* Newbury Park, CA: Sage.

Boruch, R. F., & Cecil, J. S. (1979). *Assuring the confidentiality of social research data.* Philadelphia: University of Pennsylvania Press.

Boruch, R. F., & Wothke, W. (Eds.). (1985). *Randomization and field experimentation.* San Francisco: Jossey-Bass.

Datta, L. E., & Perloff, R. (Eds.). (1979). *Improving evaluations.* Beverly Hills, CA: Sage.

DiClemente, R. J., & Peterson, J. L. (Eds.). (1994). *Preventing AIDS: Theories and methods of behavioral interventions.* New York: Plenum Press.

Fitz-Gibbon, C. T., & Morris, L. L. (1987). *How to design a program evaluation.* Newbury Park, CA: Sage.

Goetz, J. P., & LeCompte, M. D. (1984). *Ethnography and qualitative design in educational research.* New York: Academic Press.

King, J. A., Morris, L. L., & Fitz-Gibbon, C. T. (1987). *How to assess program implementation.* Beverly Hills: Sage.

Kosecoff, J., & Fink, A. (1982). *Evaluation basics-a practitioner's manual.* Beverly Hills: Sage.

McKillip, J. (1987). *Needs analysis. Tool for the human services and education.* Newbury Park, CA: Sage.

Miles, M. B., & Huberman, A. M. (1994). *Qualitative data analysis* (2nd ed., pp. 1–15). Thousand Oaks, CA: Sage.

Morgan, D. L. (1988). *Focus groups as qualitative research.* Newbury Park, CA: Sage.

Morgan, D. L. (Ed.). (1993). *Successful focus groups. Advancing the state of the art.* Newbury Park, CA: Sage.

Morris, L. L., Fitz-Gibbon, C. T., & Freeman, M. E. (1987). *How to communicate evaluation findings.* Newbury Park, CA: Sage.

Patton, M. (1986). *Utilization-focused evaluation.* Beverly Hills, CA: Sage.

Patton, M. Q. (1980). *Qualitative evaluation methods.* Beverly Hills, CA: Sage.

Sechrest, L. (1985). Evaluating health care. *American Behavioral Scientist, 28,* 527–542.

Sechrest, L., West, S. G., Phillips, M. A., Redner, R., & Yeaton, W. (1979). Some neglected problems in evaluation research: Strength and integrity of treatments. In L. Sechrest *et al.* (Eds.), *Evaluation studies review annual* (vol. 4, pp. 15–35). Beverly Hills, CA: Sage.

Shadish, W. R., Jr., Cook, T. D., & Leviton, L. C. (1991). Foundations of program evaluation. Newbury Park, CA: Sage.

Sisk, J. E., Hewitt, M., & Metcalf, K. L. (1988). The effectiveness of AIDS education. *Health Affairs, 7,* 37–51.

Soriano, F. I. (1995). *Conducting needs assessments: A multidisciplinary approach.* Thousand Oaks, CA: Sage.

Stecher, B. M., & Davis, W. A. (1987). *How to focus an evaluation.* Newbury Park, CA: Sage.

Stewart, D. W., & Shamdasani, P. N. (1990). *Focus groups. Theory and practice.* Newbury Park, CA: Sage.

Strauss, A., & Corbin, J. (1990). *Basics of qualitative research.* Newbury Park, CA: Sage.

Thomas, S. B., Chen, M. S., & So'Brien Van Putten, J. M. (1991). A program planning manual and evaluation manual for HIV education programs: A primer for ethnic and racial minority community based organizations. Columbus, OH: Ohio Department of Health.

US Conference of Mayors. (1990, April). *Focus groups: Process for developing HIV education materials, HIV Education Case Studies,* No. 2, pp. 1–24.

US Conference of Mayors. (1992, September). Proposal writing for HIV/AIDS prevention grants. *HIV/AIDS Program Technical Assistance Reports* (pp. 1–16).

Webb, E. J., Campbell, D. T., Schwartz, R. D., & Sechrest, L. (1966). *Unobtrusive measures: Nonreactive research in the social sciences*. Chicago: Rand MacNally College Publishing.

Windsor, R., Baranowski, T., Clark, N., & Cutter, G. (1984). *Evaluation of health promotion and education programs*. Mountain View, CA: Mayfield.

Winett, R. A., King, A. C., & Altman, D. G. (1989). *Health psychology and public health*. New York: Pergamon.

Yeaton, W. H., & Sechrest, L. (1987). No-difference research. In D. S. Corray, H. S. Bloom, & R. J. Light, (Eds.), *Evaluation practice in review: New directions for program evaluation*, (No. 34, pp. 67–82). San Francisco: Jossey-Bass.

About the Authors

JOANNE E. MANTELL received a Masters of Science degree in Public Health in 1977 and a Doctor of Philosophy in Public Health in 1982 from the University of California at Los Angeles, School of Public Health, Division of Behavioral Sciences and Health Education. She also holds a Masters of Science from Columbia University, School of Social Work. Prior to becoming involved in AIDS work in 1985, she conducted social–psychological research on support networks and coping with cancer.

Dr. Mantell is currently a consultant working at the HIV Center for Clinical and Behavioral Studies at the New York State Psychiatric Institute, Psychosocial and Qualitative Assessment Core, and Medical and Health Research Association of New York City, Inc. Dr. Mantell also is a lecturer at Columbia University, School of Public Health, Division of Sociomedical Sciences, where she has taught courses in program evaluation and women and AIDS.

She served as principal investigator of the behavioral research program through a Cooperative Agreement (#U62/CCU201065) awarded to Gay Men's Health Crisis (GMHC) from the US Centers for Disease Control (CDC) (1986–1988). She was also the Principal Investigator of a CDC Cooperative Agreement (#U62/CCU203330) on Prevention of Perinatal Transmission (1988–1994) and a National Institute on Drug Abuse grant (R-01 DA05995) on Promoters and Barriers to HIV Testing and Risk Reduction among Inner-City Women: The Cultural Network Project (1990–1994). Both of these projects were administered through Medical and Health Research Association of New York City, Inc. in collaboration with the New York City Department of Health. Dr. Mantell also served on a Health Services Improvement Fund Committee to assist community-based organizations in their efforts to evaluate AIDS prevention programs.

Dr. Mantell spent 9 months in 1995–1996 as a consultant to the South African Department of Health's HIV/AIDS and STD Programme. Combining her interests in HIV and reproductive health, she developed an implementation plan and a health care worker training program for the introduction of female barrier methods into public health clinics. She has written numerous articles in the area of AIDS prevention and research and is currently completing a book on women and AIDS with several of her colleagues.

ANTHONY T. DiVITTIS received a Masters of Arts degree in Clinical Psychology from Indiana University of Pennsylvania in 1980. He is a doctoral candidate in Psychometrics, Department of General Experimental Psychology, at Fordham University in New York.

Prior to his involvement in AIDS research in 1986, Mr. DiVittis was part of the Internal Evaluation Team assessing the impact of a Title III grant at Baruch College of the City University of New York. He was also an adjunct instructor at Baruch in the

Department of Statistics and Computer Information Systems. He has served as the statistician on a National Institute of Mental Health-funded psychiatric study at Cornell University Medical Center at the Payne Whitney Clinic. Mr. DiVittis was the first research director at Gay Men's Health Crisis for the CDC-funded project Prevention of HIV Transmission: AIDS Risk-Reduction with High-Risk Groups from 1986 to 1988. From 1988 to 1990, he served as cohort coordinator, New York City Department of Health, AIDS Research Unit, on the CDC-funded Prevention of Perinatal HIV Transmission Project. From 1990 to 1991, Mr. DiVittis was the project director on the CDC-funded Northern Brooklyn Partner Study (#U64/CCU203274).

Currently, he is a senior health care program planner analyst at Woodhull Medical and Mental Health Center in Brooklyn, New York, where he is grants and data manager for the AIDS Center Program. He currently manages nine New York State and federally funded HIV/AIDS service grants and is the training coordinator for homeless residents in shelters, wherein training enables participants to become peer educators and outreach workers. He has worked as a consultant to the US Conference of Mayors' Community-Based Initiative. As a volunteer for the Hyacinth Foundation, Mr. DiVittis has run support groups for gay men with HIV disease and has served on the Hudson County Community Advisory Council, in Jersey City, New Jersey. He currently is the co-principal investigator of an evaluation of the Ryan White HIV/AIDS Dental Reimbursement Program, funded by the Health Resources and Services Administration, with Dr. Mantell.

MARILYN I. AUERBACH received a Masters of Public Health in 1979 and a Doctorate of Public Health in 1989 from Columbia University, School of Public Health, Management and Policy Division. She also has a Masters of Science Degree in Library Science from the University of Michigan. Dr. Auerbach has held education and research positions at Planned Parenthood Federation, Inc., New York Hospital–Cornell University Medical Center, and Columbia University School of Public Health. From 1990 to 1993 she was an evaluation consultant to the Cornell University Medical Center for an AIDS education and training program funded by the National Institute of Mental Health.

For the past 10 years, she has worked in the Community Health Education Program, Hunter College School of Health Sciences, City University of New York, where she is an assistant professor and the director of the Community Health Education Program. She has worked closely with institutions and community-based organizations to facilitate students' application of theory in practice. For the past 12 years, she has been a volunteer at GMHC. Dr. Auerbach has taught at the graduate and undergraduate level, with emphasis on community assessment, evaluation, and policy. She has been recently appointed deputy chair of the Sexual Harassment Committee at Hunter College.

Her publications have been in the areas of AIDS, community-based health promotion intervention, and reproductive health education. Dr. Auerbach has held offices at the local and national levels in the Society for Public Health Education and the American Public Health Association. Currently, she serves on the board of the Public Health Association of New York City.

Author Index

Subject Index